Treating AIDS

Treating AIDS

Politics of Difference, Paradox of Prevention

THURKA SANGARAMOORTHY

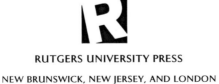

RUTGERS UNIVERSITY PRESS

NEW BRUNSWICK, NEW JERSEY, AND LONDON

LIBRARY OF CONGRESS CATALOGING-IN-PUBLICATION DATA

Sangaramoorthy, Thurka, 1975–

Treating AIDS : politics of difference, paradox of prevention / Thurka Sangaramoorthy.

pages cm

Includes bibliographical references and index.

ISBN 978–0–8135–6373–2 (hardcover : alk. paper)—ISBN 978–0–8135–6374–9
(e-book)

1. AIDS (Disease)—Social aspects. 2. Health services accessibility—United States.
3. Social status—Health aspects—United States. 4. Haitians—United States—Social
conditions. I. Title.

RA643.8.S225 2014

362.19697′92—dc23   2013027188

A British Cataloging-in-Publication record for this book
is available from the British Library.

Visit our website: http://rutgerspress.rutgers.edu

Manufactured in the United States of America

For my parents, with deepest gratitude

CONTENTS

FIGURES AND TABLES

Figures

Tables

ACKNOWLEDGMENTS

The process of completing this book was a long labor of love, hard work, and personal sacrifice. Although at times it was an intensely lonely and isolating practice, it could not have been completed without the love and support of many people. I wish to convey my enormous gratitude to those who have played an important role in the formulation and completion of this journey.

Much of this work was inspired by scholars at the Joint Medical Anthropology Program at the University of California, San Francisco and Berkeley, who taught me to think and act in ways that I never dreamed possible. I am particularly thankful to Vincanne Adams, who has always pushed me to think beyond the levels of conventional theoretical paradigms, for providing such valuable advice long after my formal studies ended. I would like to thank Yewoubdar Beyene, Sharon Kaufman, and Edwina Newsom for ensuring that funding was available for this research and for providing much-needed support after the untimely death of Gay Becker.

My growth as a scholar and a person would not have been possible without the late Gay Becker. Her intelligence, unwavering support, and positive attitude was always a source of strength for me. Her passion and dedication to her research and lifework closely mirrored her conduct as a mentor. In other words, she was the same person both inside and outside the classroom, in and out of the research context. She was an exceptional person who devoted a great deal of thought and time to others. My gratitude and admiration for her is beyond words.

In addition, I am highly indebted to Philippe Bourgois. His astute recognition of the problems of ethnographic research has taught me to become a better scholar and, more important, a critically engaged person in the world. Furthermore, he has steadfastly reminded me of the importance of voicing my own reservations and struggles in bringing seemingly disparate theoretical strands of scholarship together. Without his support, I would not have been as confident in asserting the benefits of dialogue between studies in public health, science and technology studies, and critical medical anthropology.

Charis Thompson also provided invaluable support as teacher and guide. She always made me feel comfortable and normal whenever I doubted myself, and she gave me the encouragement to move forward whenever I felt stuck.

No one has played as great a role in inspiring this work as Charles Briggs. Although our relationship began as a leap of faith toward the very end of my fieldwork in South Florida, his intellectual vision and rigor motivated me to think and work beyond what I thought were the limits of my abilities. His brilliance never kept him from being an exceptional teacher and friend, and his astute understanding of the complexities of my research continually inspires me to work and think harder. I will always be thankful for his generous and unwavering support and friendship.

Likewise, in Miami, I would like to thank those with whom I worked at the Haitian Summer Institute at Florida International University, particularly Jacques Pierre. My research could not have progressed nearly as well as it did without my institutional affiliation with the University of Miami and the informal discussions I had with J. Bryan Page and Edward LiPuma. Most of all, I am thankful for the mentorship of Louis H. Marcelin at the University of Miami. His limitless support helped me get my foot in many doors, and his intellectual and methodological rigor alleviated the many struggles that I encountered during fieldwork in Miami and with various Haitian communities. In addition, for the first time in my life, I was able to speak honestly with an anthropologist who, like me, confronts the daily realities of being a racial and ethnic minority in a discipline that often turns a blind eye to its past and continuing legacies of marginalization. His strength, humility, and perseverance personally and professionally in the face of hardship has been a true inspiration in all aspects of my life.

I must also mention how much my life and work have been deeply enriched by Ben Hickler, Ippolytos Kalofonos, Jennifer Liu, and Betsy Pohlman. They have given and continue to give me the kind of intimate support that only people in the same situation can do. I am deeply indebted to them and others, including Alex Choby, Johanna Crane, Beverly Davenport, Robin Higashi, Saida Hodzic, Seth Holmes, Yoshiko Konishi, and Simon Lee, for all the years of intellectual stimulation and hearty laughter. Likewise, Kristin Bright, Lauren Fordyce, Richard Giosio, and Suzanne Carroll Woodard provided me with invaluable friendship throughout my fieldwork in Miami.

I also want to thank Peter Brown, Svea Closser, Douglas Feldman, David Malebranche, and Ann Russ, who welcomed me as a colleague and helped in the writing process during my years in Atlanta and Rochester, New York. I am particularly indebted to the cohorts of students from my Anthropology of Global HIV/AIDS seminar at Emory University's Global Health, Culture, and Society program. During a time when I felt disheartened about the future of HIV/AIDS research in governmental public health agencies, these young people inspired me in many ways. Thank you for your collegiality, intense curiosity, and unfettered idealism. Although you may have not have known it, you made me fall in love with my work again.

I am also indebted to colleagues at the Centers for Disease Control and Prevention (CDC), particularly those at the National Center for HIV/AIDS, Viral Hepatitis, Sexually Transmitted Diseases, and Tuberculosis Prevention. To say that my time at the CDC was a life-changing experience would be an understatement. I began my three-year tenure there with the expectation of infusing ethnography into public health prevention methods. I soon realized that I needed to start the conversation at an earlier stage, beginning with the usefulness of mixed methods before moving on to qualitative or ethnographic work. Spending an enormous amount of time in long daily meetings, writing administrative reports, and conceptualizing policy papers often seemed overwhelming and pointless at the time, but I realize now how much this experience has added to my life, both personally and professionally. I want to thank Fred Bloom, Mahnaz Charania, Hazel Dean, Audrey Dowling, Kevin Fenton, Jessie Ford, Zanetta Gant, Kathleen McDavid Harrison, Matthew Hogben, Megan Ivankovich, David Johnson, William E. Jones, Yzette Lanier, Tanya LeBlanc, Penny Loosier, Reshma Mahendra, Donna McCree, Eleanor McLellan, Greg Millett, Ramal Moonesinghe, Ranell Myles, Thomas Painter, Laurie C. Reid, Karen Resha, Rebecca Schmidt, Sonia Singh, Angela M. Smith, Madeleine Sutton, Bindu Tharian, Jo Valentine, Petra Vallila-Buchman, Mary Vernon-Smiley, Mikel Walters, and Samantha Williams for teaching me a tremendous amount about the true meaning of collaboration and partnerships. I have learned a great deal about how to think practically, speak and write clearly, and work with various constituents and within the constraints of severely limited resources. I appreciate and will apply these valuable lessons in various aspects of my life.

I want to single out a few people at the CDC in particular. First, I am indebted to Karen Kroeger and Kim Williams for the endless guidance and support that they have given me. Karen taught me by example how to be an effective anthropologist in the rough seas of public health at governmental agencies, and Kim modeled the virtues of patience, humility, and perseverance in the face of incessant expectations and rigid deadlines. I want to thank Eleanor Fleming, Tracey Hardy, and Puja Seth for their friendship and the many tears and laughter that we have shared together. I will always cherish our time together.

At the University of Maryland, College Park, I am grateful for the Department of Anthropology's continued support. Thank you for giving me the freedom to write.

I want to express my sincere gratitude to my writing partners for the past two years: Adia Benton and Jennifer Liu. Without their support, guidance, and friendship, this manuscript would not be where it is today. Thank you for seeing things that I did not and for pushing me to think of my work as a useful intervention. I look forward to many years of working together.

This study would not have been possible without the generous institutional and financial support of the National Institute on Aging and the National Institute on Minority Health and Health Disparities at the National Institutes of Health, the Association of Prevention Teaching and Research, the Oak Ridge Institute for Science and Education, Sigma Xi, USA Funds Access to Education, the US Department of Education's Foreign Language and Area Studies Program, and the University of California, San Francisco.

I am indebted to Peter Mickulas for seeing this book through to publication and to the rest of the helpful staff at of Rutgers University Press. The comments I received from external reviewers and copyeditors were extremely valuable and helped make the narrative more accessible to a wider audience. I would also like to thank the Taylor & Francis Group for the permission to expand on my article "Treating the Numbers: HIV/AIDS Surveillance, Subjectivity, and Risk," in *Medical Anthropology* 31 (4) (2012).

Most important, I am humbled by the generosity of spirit of the people who allowed me into their lives in Miami. It is never easy to have a stranger hanging around, trying to insert herself into one's daily routine, and I am very thankful to the many men and women who shared their stories of struggle and joy with me. Although their names must remain anonymous for reasons of confidentiality, they are by no means nameless or anonymous in my thoughts and gratitude. I am particularly grateful to three wonderful women who wish to remain anonymous, who took me into their lives and treated me like a daughter. Anthropological fieldwork can be isolating, but I always stayed focused and grounded through the familial relationships that these women provided. Their gratitude, humor, and love for life through some of the most tragic situations I have ever witnessed put things into proper perspective and taught me life lessons that I could not have possibly learned in government offices or ivory towers.

I am also indebted to Eddie Jean Baptiste, Marlene Bastien, Frank Dardompre, Stanley Denis, Hudes Desrameaux, Katiana Diaz, Jeline Fertil, Leoni Hermatin, Dushyantha T. Jayaweera, Marie D. Jervais, Ketty Ledan, Regine Lefevre, Georges Metellus, Gepsie Mettelus, Christina Morrow, Francis Penha, Juan Carlos Riascos, Kwesi Rose, Marie Saintus, Kira Villamizar, and countless others working to better the lives of Haitians everywhere. Their tireless dedication to improving the lives of so many people who live in despair and destitution is truly remarkable, and their deep understanding of the problems of public health interventions forced me to reexamine the limits of my own questions and to rearticulate new intellectual boundaries.

This book would not have been possible without support from my immediate and extended family and friends. Thank you for cheering me on from the sidelines and for putting up with my inability to keep in better touch. I am most indebted to my husband, James Cerwinski, who has endured the many years of incessant drama that comes with my involvement in the academy. It is not easy to prioritize a partner's research, writing, and teaching needs in the face of the daily struggles that come with an equally demanding career, unexpected economic challenges, raising two children, and a cross-country move. But he did it all with endless patience and humor. I also would like to thank the two other most important people in my life, Gyan and Ashok, for putting up with a mother who is still trying her best to negotiate shifting priorities. Your endless energy and curiosity inspire me every day. I am so excited to watch you learn, grow, and explore the world.

Finally, my parents, Nala and Kathirethamby Sangaramoorthy, deserve a special note of gratitude. Almost thirty years ago, they miraculously managed to leave Sri Lanka days before the Colombo riots with about a hundred dollars in their pockets. They left relatives, livelihoods, and material belongings behind in order to begin a new life for their children. They worked around the clock, sacrificing their own educational and professional dreams to give their daughters a chance at something better. Their achievements are mine, and mine are theirs.

Treating AIDS

1

Treating Us, Treating Them

Standing on the outdoor platform of the Metrorail stop at the University of Miami on a blisteringly hot day, I was struck by a large black, white, and red poster (see figure 1.1). The poster depicted numerous celebrities, scientists, political leaders, and social activists standing and walking barefoot in graduated rows of concrete blocks. Nelson Mandela, Archbishop Desmond Tutu, Alicia Keys, Elton John, Will Smith, Zackie Achmat, and Elizabeth Taylor, among others, were shown stepping into cement and leaving a footprint—a metaphor for their commitment to the global fight against HIV/AIDS.[1] But the familiar faces were not what drew me to the poster. I was captivated by the message "we all have AIDS," which was written in large white and red capital letters across the bodies of those pictured. A much smaller phrase in the lower left corner completed the message: "if one of us does." "We all have AIDS" dwarfed both the final phrase and the human images.

I saw this sign repeatedly for several months in early 2006 in Miami's Metrorail system. The poster, it turned out, was part of what was reportedly the largest public service multimedia campaign about HIV/AIDS ever launched in the United States. The initiative was a collaborative effort between the fashion designer Kenneth Cole, chairman of the American Foundation for AIDS Research (amfAR), and KnowAIDS, a multimedia campaign funded by the Henry J. Kaiser Family Foundation, Viacom, and the CBS Corporation. The KnowAIDS campaign was a multiyear public service messaging initiative started in 2003 to "educate the general population about the impact of AIDS globally, and to promote prevention and testing among higher-risk populations, including young people, African Americans, Latinos, women, and men who have sex with men" (PRNewswire 2003).

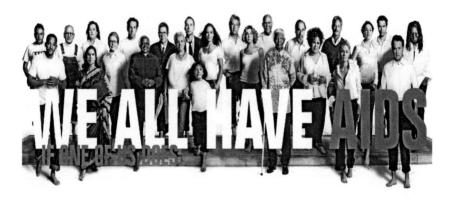

FIGURE 1.1 "We All Have AIDS" public service announcement print and outdoor advertisement commemorating World AIDS Day 2005. Kenneth Cole Productions, Inc. Used with kind permission.

The "We All Have AIDS" campaign, as it is called, built on the momentum of KnowAIDS. To raise awareness of the damaging effects of stigma in the prevention and eradication of HIV/AIDS, the campaign used print, outdoor, radio, and online advertising depicting leaders in entertainment, politics, and science standing in solidarity with those affected by HIV/AIDS. AmfAR describes the campaign as "a powerful display of the unity and solidarity we all share with the 40 million men, women, and children living with HIV/AIDS around the world" (American Foundation for AIDS Research 2006, 1). In speaking specifically about the people depicted in the ads, Kenneth Cole states: "With help from these extraordinary role models we hope to foster solidarity so that the world can focus on improving HIV prevention and treatment programs, and support necessary AIDS research" (American Foundation for AIDS Research 2006, 9). In addition to the public service announcements and media outreach, the campaign ran print advertisements in magazines such as *Vogue* and *Rolling Stone* and sold $35 limited-edition "We all have AIDS" T-shirts—products well out of reach of millions of people living with HIV/AIDS—in upscale stores such as Barneys New York and Selfridges, in London.

By calling attention to unified responsibility and the global response to HIV/AIDS, the campaign and its messages and sponsors serve as powerful tropes for recent transformations in global politics, economic consumerism, and biomedical and technological advances. The campaign marks the remarkable coming together of diverse individuals, institutions, and interests. Industry leaders in biotechnology, science, entertainment, and politics along with the fashion industry, international nonprofits, private foundations, and multibillion-dollar corporations collaborate to portray a unified front in fighting HIV/AIDS around the world. The multimedia campaign focuses on leaders and experts, referred to as "extraordinary role models," and their "unity and solidarity" with those who are living with HIV/AIDS. Those who are depicted as "higher-risk populations" or the "40 million men, women, and children living with HIV/AIDS around the world" are not the targets of the campaign. It is aimed at us, the "general population." We become the visual and material consumers of this campaign, aligning ourselves with these leaders and activists, sympathizing with those afflicted with HIV/AIDS, and buying $35 T-shirts at high-end retailers. The campaign calls on us to "have" HIV/AIDS even though we do not directly experience the debilitating physical, emotional, economic, and social consequences of HIV/AIDS.

People, Pathology, and Place

Who are the "40 million men, women, and children living with HIV/AIDS around the world"? Current HIV/AIDS research in the United States indicates that both new AIDS cases and HIV infections continue to rise exponentially among racial and ethnic minority populations (Black AIDS Institute 2011; Cargill and Stone 2005; Centers for Disease Control and Prevention 2007b, 2013a; Kaiser Family Foundation 2013; Prejean et al. 2011). These disproportionately high rates are especially pronounced in Florida, and HIV/AIDS has had a profound impact on both the state as a whole and on Miami. Florida has the third highest number of cumulative AIDS cases and the second highest number of new HIV infections in the nation, while Miami ranks third among metropolitan areas reporting cumulative AIDS cases and new HIV diagnoses (Centers for Disease Control and Prevention 2013a). In 2011, blacks[2] made up 15 percent of the adult population of Florida but accounted for 55 percent of adult AIDS cases and 48 percent of adult HIV infections reported in the state (Florida Department of Health 2011a). The annual case rate of AIDS diagnoses for blacks in Florida in 2010 was 88.5 per 100,000 people, which is much higher than the comparable figure for blacks in the United States as a whole (53.4 per 100,000) (Kaiser Family Foundation 2011). In 2010 HIV/AIDS was the fourth leading cause of death for black adults living in Florida; it had been the leading cause of death from 1988 until 2010 (Florida Department of Health 2010).

Miami plays a key role in the national debates about HIV/AIDS prevention and intervention because it is a place where relations between race, ethnicity, risk, and HIV/AIDS are continually evolving. Growing concerns about disparities in HIV/AIDS rates among blacks and Hispanics have brought discourses of race and ethnicity to the fore.[3] Many scholars and public health experts argue that existing HIV/AIDS prevention strategies, which are focused on testing, treatment, education initiatives, and interventions designed to change people's behavior, fail to work in communities of color because they are not culturally appropriate (Marcelin and Marcelin 2001; Marcelin et al. 2006; Martin et al. 1995; Needle et al. 2003; D. Williams and Jackson 2000). They also claim that grouping together Miami's numerous different ethnic groups into a few labels such as "black" or "Hispanic" obscures specific risks that prevent the successful formulation of research and community-based preventive intervention strategies (Marcelin et al. 2006; Norris and DeMarco 2004). They advocate for the standard use of more-nuanced racial and ethnic categories such as "Haitian," even though significant demographic changes, public debates and movements, and recent advances in genetic research have increasingly called into question biological distinctions between races.

The category of "Haitian" and its link to pathology and HIV/AIDS are particularly salient for Haitians in Miami and for health and social service providers and advocates who work with Haitians. In the early 1980s, at the beginning of the HIV/AIDS epidemic, the Centers for Disease Control and Prevention and many public health officials in other US agencies identified Haitians as one of the four high-risk groups—infamously dubbed the "4-H club" because of its inclusion of homosexuals, hemophiliacs, heroin users, and Haitians—and in 1990 the Food and Drug Administration prohibited anyone of Haitian descent from donating blood in the United States. These actions of classifying and labeling an entire national group as high risk and placing all of its members among those whose so-called immoral behaviors placed them at risk for acquiring HIV/AIDS fueled preexisting racial tensions and led to various acts of violence and large-scale discrimination against Haitian emigrants (Fairchild and Tynan 1994; Farmer 1992; Nachman 1993). The direct official association of Haitians with HIV/AIDS, although later repealed, caused and still causes severe consequences for Haitians around the world. The collection of Haitian-specific HIV/AIDS data also continues to be a highly debated issue in places like Miami because of this legacy.

Data about HIV/AIDS rates for Haitians at the local, state, and national levels are very scarce. The Florida Department of Health (2011b) does collect statistics on Haitians, and 2011 estimates—the most recent available—are that the Haitian-born population comprised 2 percent of the population but 7 percent of the HIV/AIDS population and 16 percent of the black HIV/AIDS population in the state.[4] Experts stress that these estimates are gross undercounts due to Haitians' unstable patterns of housing, high mobility, distrust of government in general and health officials in particular, immigration status, and other factors (Marcelin and Marcelin 2001; Stepick and Stepick 1990). In addition, the anthropologists Louis Marcelin and Louise Marcelin (2001) claim that county health officials began to estimate new HIV/AIDS cases only in 1999, and annual reports since then reveal that Haitians account for 11–12 percent of all new cases of HIV/AIDS, the highest of the groups in the "black/African-American" category.

A majority of these cases (80 percent) were found during mandatory blood tests for adjustment of immigration status, and not as a result of effective surveillance or voluntary testing (Marcelin and Marcelin 2001).

Why Don't We All Have HIV/AIDS?

There is an inherently powerful and complex paradox underlying the science and practice of HIV/AIDS prevention, which is embodied both by the "We All Have AIDS" campaign's focus on collective advocacy mobilized to combat HIV/AIDS around the globe and by the staggeringly disproportionate rates of HIV/AIDS in many places, like Miami. HIV/AIDS prevention makes claims about the universal impact of HIV/AIDS and the ensuing social responsibility that we all have through national multimedia campaigns like "We All Have AIDS." At the same time, HIV/AIDS prevention efforts focus on "higher-risk populations" and divide groups of people through the use of categories of social difference—that is, race, ethnicity, sexual orientation, and national origin. Although many diverse groups and interests come together in global HIV/AIDS prevention to promote the universality of HIV/AIDS as a social, political, economic, and biomedical problem, in places like Miami, developments in HIV/AIDS prevention are rooted in and focused exclusively on disparities in HIV/AIDS morbidity and mortality framed by the rubrics of race, ethnicity, and nationality.

In this book, I am concerned with how a unified responsibility to global HIV/AIDS exists alongside the uncontested presence of severe disparities in HIV/AIDS rates, treatment, and stigma. I am interested not only in how we all have HIV/AIDS, but also in how we come to have HIV/AIDS and the ways in which social difference firmly structures our experiences and management of HIV/AIDS. I examine this paradox by documenting an on-the-ground view of HIV/AIDS prevention programs in Miami and their effect on the health and well-being of Haitians, a transnational community long plagued by the stigma of being HIV/AIDS carriers.

This book addresses three central questions. First, how does a universal responsibility for HIV/AIDS around the globe operate in conjunction with the indisputable existence of disparities in HIV/AIDS rates? Second, how are categories of social difference—particularly race and ethnicity—produced, sustained, and transformed by HIV/AIDS prevention science and practice? Finally, how does HIV/AIDS prevention work in the Haitian community, given its long history of discrimination and its distrust of public health and social institutions?

These questions are best answered using highly interdisciplinary theoretical and methodological frameworks. By focusing on cultural interpretations of marginalized populations or the political economy of HIV/AIDS in Miami, I might come to understand how social vulnerability is experienced and enacted in Miami or how larger geopolitical forces affect individual suffering.

But by critically engaging with and integrating theoretical and methodological approaches from medical anthropology, epidemiology, science and technology studies, critical race theory, and citizenship, I am able to examine thoroughly how the health and well-being of individuals and groups are affected by larger social formations, cultural norms, and local and global politics. By working in key sites of HIV/AIDS scientific and policy governance, prevention programs, and the social worlds of Haitians living in Miami, I can interpret more broadly the ways in which HIV/AIDS prevention reproduces and naturalizes categories of social difference and fails to capture the reality of the daily lives of the people it tries to know and act on.

Universality and Fragmentation

Based on long-term ethnographic fieldwork, I chronicle how HIV/AIDS prevention is a critical framework through which we can observe the paradox of postmodernity (Harvey 1989), in which there is both a celebration of fragmentation as well as an embrace of unification (or globalization) in an increasingly transnational and commodity-driven world. Recent innovations in science and technology, such as molecular genetics and evidence-based medicine, have transformed the ways in which we come to see and understand the conceptualization of life itself, from our universal human identity to the vast disparities and inequities that infiltrate all aspects of our society (Clarke et al. 2003; Dumit 2003; Franklin and Lock 2003; Lock et al. 2000; Rabinow 1999; Rose 1999, 2007; Thompson 2005). A paradigm shift in the provision of health—from the diagnosis and treatment of disease through clinical mediation to the emphasis on risk factor analyses and prevention—has also ensued because of these broader changes in life and labor. The science and practice of HIV/AIDS prevention, for example, focus on specific personal behavioral risk factors and concentrate primarily on obtaining explanations for differentials in HIV/AIDS rates at the level of individual variation (Parker 2001). Although social and structural factors have been slowly incorporated into broader public health discourses, variations based on social differences (such as race, ethnicity, culture, and nationality) and individual behavioral traits (for example, having sex with men, for men, and the use of intravenous drugs, for everyone) have become synonymous with risk factors that increase vulnerability to HIV/AIDS. In HIV/AIDS prevention, categories of social difference and behavioral risk have become essential components of how we come to understand, embody, and act on these broader transformations in governance and personhood.

These transformations demonstrate that HIV/AIDS prevention in the United States is not a complete or closed system. Although HIV/AIDS prevention has had a long history in the "West," becoming what the anthropologist Stacey Leigh Pigg calls "a template of accepted facts" (2001, 481), it is far from established.[5]

I argue that there is a blind spot in the study of global HIV/AIDS that presumes that HIV/AIDS knowledge in the "West" is a unified whole and is well established and systematized. This may be how HIV/AIDS prevention knowledge travels globally (as Pigg argues), but such claims about a unified and undifferentiated "West" need to be critically challenged.

The landscape of HIV/AIDS prevention in the United States is highly fragmented, flexible, and deeply contested. Controversies and struggles about how HIV/AIDS data are interpreted, how funding should be allocated, and how HIV/AIDS prevention programs are conceived of and translated for various populations in different sites continually occur. For instance, frequent transformations in surveillance systems and enumerative methods that structure US-based HIV/AIDS prevention programs highlight the fact that the data produced from these practices do not represent universal knowledge about HIV/AIDS, risk, or populations. The shifting of priorities in HIV/AIDS prevention from individual-level behavioral interventions to those that focus on communities increasingly conflates behavioral and biological traits with culture and reconfigures notions of community. Programs focused on so-called positive living, which emphasize empowerment and personal responsibility, do not translate well for Haitians living with HIV/AIDS because they obscure issues of economic and social marginalization. Disparities in HIV/AIDS-related health outcomes, especially those related to racial and ethnic differences, continue to be treated as facts that no longer need explanation or deliberation. Paying close attention to such debates in specific sites and communities highlights how HIV/AIDS prevention in the United States is in a constant state of flux. Studying these controversies also provides new ways of thinking about economically, politically, and socially marginalized populations in the United States and how they come to interpret and refute health interventions and constructions of difference.

My work builds on the momentum of critical studies of HIV/AIDS in the United States that have focused on citizenship, globalization, and justice. Anthropology and other disciplines were remarkably unsuccessful in responding early to the epidemic,[6] and although incredible progress has been made in anthropological studies of HIV/AIDS since then, there is still much left to do. Ethnographies of US-based treatment and prevention programs from the perspective of both HIV/AIDS experts and clients still lag behind those focused on other countries. For instance, ethnographies in settings outside the United States have expanded and are investigating the social, economic, and political consequences of the epidemic in countries where it has had the greatest impact, as well as the productive and repressive role of governments and nongovernmental structures (see, for example, Beine 2003; Benton 2012; Biehl 2007; Biruk 2012; Butt and Eves 2008; Farmer 1992; Fassin 2007, 2009; Fordham 2004; Frank 2009; Gutmann 2007; Hyde 2007; Kalofonos 2010; Lockhart 2008; Lyttleton

2000; Nguyen 2005, 2010; Owczarzak 2009; Pigg 2001; Rödlach 2006; Setel 1999; Susser 2009; Thornton 2008). With some notable exceptions (see, for example, Bourgois 2000; Epstein 1996; Parker and Aggleton 2003; Patton 1985, 1990; Sangaramoorthy 2008, 2012; Treichler 1999), scholars concentrating on HIV/AIDS in the United States have not underscored these same considerations but rather continue to focus on sexuality, drug use, and racial disparities, following theoretical directions that treat culture as resulting from a range of interconnected social and structural interactions. I add to the critical studies of anthropology and global health by focusing on the multiple controversies and struggles over science, governance, and citizenship that ground HIV/AIDS prevention in the United States.

Reproducing and Naturalizing Social Difference

In this book, I also depict how medical, epidemiological, and social constructions of HIV/AIDS link pathology to racial, ethnic, and cultural identities at a time when critical debates over race, ethnicity, and citizenship continue to gain traction in scientific and public spheres. HIV/AIDS prevention programs help reinforce categories of social difference and maintain race, ethnicity, and culture as risk factors for HIV/AIDS through everyday practices. Much of this is due to the nature of epidemiology—which is the dominant way of understanding risk in medical and clinical interventions—and its proclivity for reductionism, in which the individual serves as a prime unit of analysis, groups are seen as homogeneous, and race and ethnicity are assumed to be individual characteristics instead of social relations of power (Baer et al. 1997; Commission on Social Determinants of Health 2008; Cooper and David 1986; Krieger 1994; McMichael 1995; Navarro 2000, 2004; Raphael 2006).

Many scholars have investigated individual- and group-level vulnerabilities to particular diseases (Comstock et al. 2004) or how race and ethnicity constitute biomedical categorizations where intragroup variations are obscured, intergroup differences are inflated, and health inequalities attributable to social structural factors are veiled (Glick Schiller 1992; Krieger 1994; Krieger and Fee 1994). Alan Goodman (2000) and Nancy Krieger (2000a, 2000b), for instance, argue that although attributing ethnic and racial differences in disease to genetic differences is scientific racialism, the consequences of a racialized society must be tracked until the elimination of all disparities based on race and ethnicity. Others similarly contend that the concepts of race and ethnicity are social constructs and therefore too rudimentary to be useful in health disparities research; they call for explorations of the effects of racism, not race and ethnicity themselves, in causative models of health disparities (Kaufman and Cooper 2001). Still others call for a race-neutral approach of genotyping populations rather than using self-identifications based on specific racial and ethnic categories (Wood 2001).

Using race and ethnicity in health research in order to document inequality and measure the success of initiatives aimed at reducing health disparities has been and can be useful because such studies turn our attention to the increasing impact of health disparities and emphasize the importance of multifactorial models for risk (Banks et al. 2006; Centers for Disease Control and Prevention 2010; Harper et al. 2007; Hart and Williams 2009; Jones 2000; Krieger 2008; Pappas et al. 1993; Singh and Siahpush 2006). But this literature has not done enough to question the role of biomedical and public health science in the construction of categories of social difference as risk factors. We often dismiss as bad or racist science any research that reformulates concepts of genetic and biological differences among races or fabricates direct causative links among race, genetics, and disease (see, for example, Gilbert et al. 2007; Pape et al. 2007). But we are often less critically reflective about the multitude of studies that measure and document racial and ethnic disparities in health. Without questioning the legitimacy of the studies that collect racial and ethnic data for the purposes of monitoring health disparities, I argue that when we support such studies almost without question, we run the risk of relegating these approaches to idealistic notions of a pure and objective science, one that has the power to monitor the racist and ethnocentric ills of society. We need to encourage all researchers who use race and ethnicity to critically examine how these categories of social difference come to be constructed, used, and interpreted in specific social and historical contexts, and how they themselves invoke race and ethnicity in their own research and writing. HIV/AIDS prevention science does more than measure and document racial and ethnic disparities in health. Through HIV/AIDS surveillance and categorization practices, it also conflates social and biological differences and risk, making relations among race, ethnicity, and disease seem natural and reinscribing the validity and potency of racial and ethnic differences. Categories of social difference such as race and ethnicity have become foundational to how HIV/AIDS science, treatment, and prevention are administered and understood. It is only by investigating the complex and obscured social history of the naturalization of racial and ethnic disparities in health that we are able to realize how these categories of difference have come to be seen as commonsensical realities and facts that no longer need clarification, rationalization, or critical reflection.

Haitians and HIV/AIDS Prevention

Finally, I focus in this book on the specific problems facing diverse immigrant and ethnic communities and illustrate how Haitians strategically identify with various institutions and diseases in order to gain access to critical resources that are otherwise unavailable to them. For many Haitians facing social, political, and economic marginalization, HIV/AIDS represents social protection in the form of cash subsidies and free medical care, and HIV/AIDS prevention becomes the platform through which they assert claims of social membership and citizenship. Translations of HIV/AIDS prevention programming, as a result, do not occur smoothly or as planned in Haitian communities.

In Miami, Haitians are heavily affected by the HIV/AIDS epidemic; they are also blamed for the transnational spread of the disease.[7] As black migrants, Haitians face difficulties getting continuous HIV/AIDS treatment and care through public health and social welfare programs because of their high mobility, tenuous legal status, and lack of economic resources. Sadly, this is not surprising. Migration and mobility have long been key components in discussions of the HIV/AIDS epidemic and continue to contribute to the portrayal of migrants as vectors of disease (Crush et al. 2006; Fairchild and Tynan 1994; Goodwin-Gill 1996; Haour-Knipe and Rector 1996; Herdt 1997; Kuntz 1990; Portes 1997; Quinn 1994).

As noted above, at the beginning of the AIDS epidemic, Haitians were identified as a group at high risk for HIV/AIDS. This positioning of an entire nationality has had adverse effects on Haitian emigrants worldwide, especially those residing in the United States. Such classifications and labels, in spite of being partially repealed, caused a tremendous amount of discrimination against and fear of the community and instigated a plethora of anti-Haitian practices such as housing evictions and job losses (Fairchild and Tynan 1994; Farmer 1992; Nachman 1993). Reports of HIV/AIDS in Haitians still reflect widespread prejudices about Haitians as unclean and disease ridden (Farmer 1992; Farmer and Kim 1991; Marcelin 2005; Nachman 1993). As a result, many Haitian and Haitian Americans, fearful of repercussions, identified themselves as other black immigrants or as African Americans (Farmer 1992; Marcelin 2005). This practice continues today among many Haitian youths and adults as a reaction to persisting negative stereotypes of Haitians (Laguerre 1984, 1998; Marcelin 2005; Nachman 1993; Portes and Stepick 1993; Stepick 1992, 1998; Stepick et al. 2003; Zéphir 1996).

Furthermore, the long history of blame and discrimination serves to reinforce Haitian resistance and hostility toward public health educational and intervention programs (Farmer and Kim 1991). Haitian professionals, intellectuals, working-class individuals, religious groups, and leaders continue to evade any relationship to the epidemic; many face stigmatization from their communities for their association with HIV/AIDS prevention efforts (Farmer and Kim 1991; Marcelin 2005). Many Haitians who are HIV-positive take great care in hiding their illness from others. I first became aware of the extent of this issue during my final year as a master's student in public health in New York City in 2001, when I was asked to serve as a graduate intern for a prospective study assessing unmet needs and the delivery of HIV/AIDS services from the perspective of people living with HIV/AIDS in Westchester, Rockland, and Putnam Counties. The study documented, through surveys, the epidemiological profiles of the growing numbers of HIV-positive individuals living in the New York City suburbs. A senior colleague confided to me that the project was having a difficult time recruiting a significant number of Haitians and Haitian Americans through health and social service agencies, and that even though Haitians were accessing health and social services, many refused to participate in the study. After conversations with providers and clients, I found that many HIV/AIDS prevention and interventions programs, like the one for which I worked, are perceived to be accountable not to Haitian communities, but to their sponsoring institutions—the same agencies, such as the Centers for Disease Control and Prevention, whose policies and actions are deeply resented by Haitians.

Issues of mobility and political and economic marginalization, as well as historical legacies of discrimination, have a great impact on the way that information about HIV/AIDS is conceptualized, received, and put to use. In addition, in the era of globalization, citizenship is becoming framed increasingly outside of the juridical sphere of modern democratic nation-states; transnational institutions and policies exert increasing influence over practices traditionally associated with citizenship, such as rights-based protection and experiences of collective identities, encouraging individuals to protect themselves from potential biological and social harm and violation by engaging in self-management practices, acquiring expert knowledge, and claiming the rights and benefits due to them (Castles and Davidson 2000; Foucault 2000; Hann and Dunn 1996; Laguerre 1998; Ong 1999, 2003; Petryna 2002; Rose 1999; Rose and Novas 2005; Strathern 2000). At a time where shifting dynamics between rights-based politics, biology, and identity have given rise to reconfigurations of individuals as biological consumers, Haitians' struggles for political, economic, and social inclusion are rooted in the separation of citizenship and biology.

These complex issues are not addressed well, if at all, in the conceptualization and practice of HIV/AIDS programming. Providers, officials, and the public increasingly see the poor translation of HIV/AIDS interventions in Haitian communities as resulting not from social assumptions and the structural limitations of prevention programs, but from the inherent characteristics of Haitians themselves—who are viewed as racialized others who are uneducated, impoverished, and prone to high-risk behavior. In order to be effective, public health policy and programs for immigrants and highly mobile populations such as migrants must take into account how issues of mobility, immigration policy, racism, and citizenship affect those populations' vulnerability to poor health outcomes and quality of life (Sangaramoorthy and Kroeger 2013). We must consider how HIV/AIDS programs are based on policies and practices of inclusion and exclusion, and how HIV/AIDS becomes a way for Haitians, as stigmatized, racialized, and marginalized noncitizen subjects, to seek material benefits and social inclusion. At a time marked by severe global recession, political unrest, massive migration, and rising health care costs, we must reconceptualize how we come to understand HIV/AIDS so that we can offer practical solutions that can be applied beyond academia to address the limitations of public health and biomedicine.

The Dynamics of Place and Position

HIV/AIDS prevention is highly complex and interdisciplinary and occurs across multiple interrelated sites. In order to explore the paradox of HIV/AIDS prevention and its impact on social categories of difference and the Haitian community, I trace how information and knowledge about HIV/AIDS prevention science and practice circulate, traveling from sites of surveillance and regulation to various clinics and hospitals and then to the social worlds of Haitian immigrants. During fifteen months, in July 2004 and from July 2005 through August 2006, I collected various types of data including participant observation notes, transcripts of interviews with fifty-three key informants,[8] and epidemiological and surveillance data, which I define as multiple forms of information related to health, disease, and well-being that are continuously gathered for the specific purpose of monitoring population health. To demonstrate that HIV/AIDS prevention programs reinforce categories of individual and collective difference and maintain them as risk factors for HIV/AIDS, I worked closely with HIV/AIDS experts, public officials, and Haitian community members. I was able to participate and observe at multiple sites, including sites of surveillance where key aspects of HIV/AIDS prevention were determined,[9] clinical sites where HIV/AIDS prevention was implemented,[10] and the social worlds of Haitians and their social and health services providers where HIV/AIDS prevention was interpreted and acted on.[11] Using multilayered interdisciplinary approaches, I also observed and participated in the flows of knowledge, people, and practices across these sites. This sort of approach invariably requires retooling conventional methodological approaches to reflect the realities of working in highly bureaucratic and specialized sites and engaging with overstudied and virtually impenetrable groups. It also necessitates rethinking positionality and place, so that Miami is understood as an embattled global city and an essential fieldwork site for studying the paradox of HIV/AIDS prevention.

Witnessing Miami

After one long day at Miami General Hospital, I was exhausted and dreading my long commute back home. Although I had a car, I was not used to driving and often found myself taking chances on Miami's notoriously dysfunctional public transportation. Today, as luck would have it, I got off the regional Tri-Rail commuter train only to find that I just missed the bus connection to North Miami. Waiting thirty minutes for the next bus was a better option than waiting for the next train, which would not come for another hour. My bus was really quiet when I finally got on, as there were only four or five passengers on board. After another five minutes, an older black man and I were the only ones left. The driver, a middle-aged Hispanic man, suddenly pulled the bus over near a small coffee shop to get coffee and informed me that he would be back in two minutes. He didn't address the older gentleman, who was standing directly in his line of sight. In fact, he didn't even look at him. Instead he craned his head and twisted his body to look at me, even though I was sitting farther back, on the opposite side of the bus. The older man had been standing by the door as if he were about to get off, and I felt terrible that the bus driver had decided to take a coffee break without letting him off first. But the older man didn't say a single word to the driver or to me. He just sat down on the seat opposite mine, looked at his watch, pressed his lips together, and waited.

The bus driver emerged with a small styrofoam cup full of café cubano, an espresso drink sweetened with demerara sugar, and tiny plastic cups that looked like thimbles. He looked at me and asked if I wanted some coffee. I had never had café cubano, so I walked up to him, and he poured a small quantity into one of the small cups and handed it to me. I offered the older man some. He tilted his head back, laughed, and shook his head to say no. The coffee had a sweet, tan, frothy top layer, with dark strong espresso below. I sipped it while the bus took off again. The old man walked to the front of the bus and said something to the bus driver in Spanish; then he got off at the next stop.[12]

Two African American women got on next, at different stops. Both sat in the front of the bus. One of the women yelled out, "Air conditioner!" as a command. I was not sure if the driver had heard her and didn't want to respond. She began shouting "Bus driver!" with increasing volume. After what seemed like an eternity, he said, "Huh?" She responded fiercely, "It's hot in here, you gotta turn the air conditioner up!" He mumbled something to her that I couldn't hear, and she angrily replied, "You tryin' to be funny?" She became upset, yelling at the top of her voice, "That's all you had to say. Shoot! You can't treat me like this! It's not those days anymore. Not no more!" The other woman and I didn't say anything. When the first woman didn't get a response from anyone on the bus, she again repeated angrily, "It's not those days anymore! You can't be telling me to get off the damn bus!"

When I arrived in Miami in 2005 to conduct long-term ethnographic field-work in HIV/AIDS, I was unsure of what to expect. Although I had been work-ing, living, and traveling in many large cities around the world for almost a decade prior to my arrival in Miami, very little classroom or on-the-job training prepared me for the latent and overt racial, ethnic, and national tensions that I frequently witnessed in Miami. These dynamics were intrinsic pieces of the social landscape and were suggestive of a broader national, ethnic, and racial discord that somehow seemed to set Miami apart from other places I had been. They were also critical to understanding the ways in which public health prevention operates in Miami and places like it.

Others have remarked on the unique assemblages related to race, ethnicity, immigration, geography, history, and gross inequalities in both health and other socioeconomic and political realms that have made Miami distinct from other cities in the United States. Miami has often been called the "City of the Future," the "American Riviera," and "Paradise Lost" (Allman 1987; Croucher 1997; Portes and Stepick 1993). Sheila Croucher writes that "Miami is a new city—a city without a long, rich history, a city not comfortably situated within established social, economic, and political traditions of the United States, a city without a firm or deeply rooted identity" (1997, 2). Alejandro Portes and Alex Stepick echo this sentiment when they declare that "Miami is not a microcosm of the American city. It never was" (1993, xi). Miami, unlike other cities, was established by wealthy entrepreneurs who hoped to attract residents and vacationers to its sunny climate and attractive coastline rather than its commercial or manufacturing potential (Allman 1987; Grenier and Stepick 1992; Portes and Stepick 1993).

Miami evolved slowly from a tourist resort to an embattled and complex city. Experts have remarked that Miami's transformation in the twentieth century was politically overdetermined; that is, its geographic proximity and economic and political connections to Latin America and the Caribbean made it a logical entry point into United States, and its close ties with Cuba, Haiti, and various other South and Central American countries have given it a major role in politics in those places (Croucher 1997; Grenier and Stepick 1992; Portes and Stepick 1993; Stepick 1998; Stepick et al. 2003).

The city's evolution began during the Cuban Revolution, as thousands of immigrants built a prosperous enclave within Miami in the early 1970s. Cuban immigrants clashed with the older, more-established southern migrant, Jewish, and African American communities because of the newcomers' political conservatism, anticommunism, and relative isolation as they built parallel but unconnected social and cultural institutions. Waves of new immigrants—Cubans from the Mariel boatlift, Haitian refugees escaping political and economic oppression, and Nicaraguan exiles fleeing the Sandinistas—have been subject to differential immigration policies. These policies have been readier to give asylum status to Cubans refugees while trying to prevent Haitian immigration and detaining those Haitians who manage to enter the country, all of which helped fashion a turbulent ethnic kaleidoscope in Miami.

Miami has the highest percentage of foreign-born residents of any city in the United States, including 50 percent more than Los Angeles and New York (Stepick et al. 2003). Most residents of Miami are recent arrivals from Latin America and the Caribbean, and the population growth rate is due more to immigration than to local birth rates, again distinguishing Miami from other US cities (Stepick 1998). This has meant that political migrations have also produced novel economic phenomena such as a dramatic increase in the labor supply, and the growth of the Cuban and other ethnic enclaves had meant additional economic opportunities—a case where politics and economics have had a synergistic effect, turning Miami into a major trade hub (Portes and Stepick 1993). As a result of immigration patterns and US foreign policy, social and racial phenomena acquire unique configurations in Miami, where a national ethnic minority—Cuban Americans—have forced a reverse acculturation, a Latinization of space and place, by substantially controlling the city's socioeconomic, symbolic, and political power (Marcelin 2005; Portes and Stepick 1993). This has led many communities within Miami to vie with each other for political and economic power. The results have sometimes been violent, with the Liberty City Riots in 1980,[13] two major racial riots in 1982 and 1989,[14] confrontations over antibilingualism legislation in 1980,[15] and a three-year economic boycott of Cuban-owned businesses starting in 1990.[16]

One major ethnic rivalry is that between Haitians and Cubans. Florida is home to the largest concentration of those reporting "Haitian" or "Haiti" as their ancestry in the United States: of the 830,000 people reporting Haitian ancestry, approximately 376,000 live in Florida (US Bureau of the Census 2010). Many scholars and activists have long challenged the inaccuracies of census-based counts for Haitians, arguing that the framing of the questions themselves (that is, asking about place of birth and ancestry) and barriers related to undocumented immigration status, language, and high mobility have led to gross undercounts (Ember et al. 2005; Laguerre 1998). Exact figures for Haitians living in Miami are also difficult to locate. In 2007 Miami-Dade County claimed, based on its informal estimates, that the number was over 100,000, even though official Census counts that were based on those reporting Haitian ancestry estimated the number to be 95,669 (Miami-Dade County Department of Planning and Zoning 2007). Local agencies and some scholars believe the number to be much higher, anywhere from 200,000 to 1,000,000 (Colin and Paperwalla 2008; Laguerre 1984).

The anthropologist Michel Laguerre (1984, 1998) has described Haitian immigration to the United States as occurring in waves that paralleled major repressive periods in Haiti. The first wave was in the 1950s and 1960s and consisted mostly of Haitian professionals fleeing the Duvalier regime,[17] as well as a few skilled laborers from the middle and lower classes who were needed to fill the vacuum left in US industries as a result of the Vietnam War. The most recent wave of Haitian immigrants, often called the "boat people," has come from more rural areas and modest backgrounds, and these new arrivals have frequently been subject to detainment and deportation.

Public opinion that recent immigrants are diseased and backward has increased discrimination and prejudice against them, and intense class differences among Haitians have contributed to more socioeconomic disparities (Stepick 1998). A 2009 American Community Survey brief reported Haitians had lower educational attainment (18 percent of Haitian men and women aged twenty-five and older had at least a bachelor's degree, compared with 28 percent of men and 27 percent of women in the total population of the United States), lower family income (the median family income for Haitians was $46,000, compared with $61,000 for the total population), higher rates of unemployment (14 percent Haitians, compared with 10 percent in the total population), and higher rates of poverty (20 percent of Haitians, compared with 14 percent of the total population) than Americans overall (US Bureau of the Census 2010). These findings parallel those in a report compiled by the Brookings Institution on the economic situation of Haitians living in Miami (Sohmer 2005). According to this report, the median household income for Haitians living in Miami-Dade County was $27,284, well below the county rate of $35,966, and that the poverty rates for Haitians in the county (30 percent) were almost double that of the county average (18 percent), with nearly one-third of all Haitian households qualifying as low income (earning below $18,000 a year). The report attributed the Haitians' disadvantages to a largely younger population coming from an impoverished country, low educational achievement, low access to federal benefits, and a high percentage of income spent on basic housing costs (Sohmer 2005).

Many argue that Haitian economic integration into Miami has been markedly different from that of other groups like the Cubans (Kretsedemas 2004; Stepick et al. 2003). Unlike Cuban and other Hispanic immigrants who have relied heavily on existing enclave economies and political networks established by earlier waves of middle-class Hispanic immigrants, Haitians have long been politically marginalized and pushed into informal economies because they have been considered unwanted refugees, illegal aliens, black minorities, and linguistic outsiders (speaking neither English nor Spanish). In South Florida, such considerations severely restrict Haitians' economic and social opportunities (Laguerre 1998; Marcelin 2005; Portes and Stepick 1993; Sohmer 2005; Stepick 1992, 1998; Stepick et al. 2003). For instance, most recent Haitian immigrants and their families reside in the inner-city neighborhoods of Miami-Dade County. Today, Little Haiti, Liberty City, Homestead, and Florida City are heavily populated by recent Haitian immigrants and are among the most economically, politically, and socially marginalized communities in Miami (Fordyce 2008;

Mooney 2009; Stepick 1998). Although economic prosperity and active political participation are increasing, Haitians in South Florida consistently struggle to overcome restrictive immigration policies, racism, poverty, and lack of access to welfare benefits (Marcelin 2005; Sohmer 2005; Stepick et al. 2003).

Miami, therefore, serves as an important case study for the debates on universality and fragmentation. Formed through social interaction and embedded in various shifting contexts of power, the multiple communities in Miami have different experiences that reveal fluid sets of global dynamics and local practices. The city itself becomes a global space in which established theories of assimilation, acculturation, and ethnicity are questioned, and social and political identities are being continually reconfigured. Thus, Miami has contemporary significance as a lens through which convergences of people, rationalities, and goods can be viewed.

Rethinking Methods, Rethinking Positionality

Participant observation and in-depth interviews, central to ethnographic methodology, allow the researcher to make detailed and documented observations of the complexity of the interactions and interrelations among people, objects, and places (Bailey 2007; Becker and Geer 1957; Fitzpatrick 1981; Geertz 1973; Kutsche 1998; Leininger 1985). But guidelines for conducting ethnographic research say very little about negotiating entry into highly specialized sites like clinics, hospitals, and health departments or into communities—such as Haitian groups in Miami—whose residents have long been suspicious of outsiders, especially those associated with research institutions and studying HIV/AIDS, generally a stigmatized topic among Haitians. Contrary to some people's perceptions, conducting fieldwork in US cities can be extremely difficult, much as it is in other global locales. In Miami, working with Haitian community organizations and their clients and investigating issues related to HIV/AIDS was as challenging as many people had predicted: I experienced numerous obstacles, including those related to access, language, and bureaucratic red tape.

Entry into field sites and access to potential informants was heavily dependent on a gatekeeper system, and I often needed to find a well-regarded individual who was able to verify and vouch for my presence and research. My affiliation with the University of Miami (UM) also gave me legitimacy as a local scholar or UM student in many of these field sites.[18]

Not all of my sites of study involved a gatekeeper or required me to demonstrate an institutional affiliation. In these instances, I negotiated entry into institutions through health educators and outreach workers—rather than high-level administrators or bureaucrats—because of their accessibility and direct contact with Haitian clients. Often, they were deeply interested in the problems I was researching and said that my concerns mirrored their own. Many were very savvy about notions of "culture," "risk," and "community" and readily invited me to participate in activities and meetings that they organized for their Haitian clients. In all instances, I followed proper protocols in protecting confidential information, including the use of pseudonyms throughout this book to present information acquired through interviews, conversations, and participant observation notes for all informants due the sensitive nature of the topics covered. I have also chosen to use pseudonyms for health and social service providers. The HIV/AIDS prevention community in Miami is fairly small, and the number of those who provide social and health services to Haitians is even smaller; it is therefore very likely that individuals in these communities could identify their colleagues or themselves in the book. Although the observations, experiences, and conversations described throughout are not secrets, many of the people that I interviewed, observed, lived, and worked with communicated and acted in ways that could have compromised their relationships with others such as colleagues, clients, supervisors, friends, and family members. There were many times, for instance, when I worked with providers who, like many of their clients, had not disclosed their HIV-positive status to colleagues, friends, or relatives. These issues, especially in the context of my fieldwork, present unique challenges. I have also restructured some individuals' descriptions when I thought that their identity, even with a pseudonym, might be too obvious. For instance, there are only a handful of clinicians who work in small health clinics that cater to Haitians and only a few Haitians who attend HIV/AIDS educational classes or are involved in intervention programs; identifying them as such would have been equivalent to naming them. For consistency, I have used first and last names in pseudonyms for all informants; however, because I am interested how expertise is constructed and how experts convey knowledge about HIV/AIDS prevention, I use "Dr." and only a last name to denote clinicians or public health researchers with a Ph.D. For other types of health and social service providers, I mention their jobs. Finally, for the same reasons mentioned above (that is, the dearth of service providers), I have used pseudonyms for all local institutions, with the exception of those associated with local and state health departments.

I had several additional problems in interviewing and recording informants. It often took long periods of time to obtain interviews with Haitian informants, some of whom I would lose contact with altogether because they moved or their phone numbers were disconnected. Several informants also declined to be interviewed, often stating that their motivations were not "political." Even though I tried to "depoliticize" my research and explain it as something that could potentially benefit them and other Haitians, this did not change their minds. In addition, many informants or potential informants wanted or expected monetary compensation for interviews that I was not authorized to give. I often tried to get around this by providing car rides, translation help, or food, but there were several times where my requests for interviews were denied because I could not offer people money. As one woman told me, "They're giving out $10 for interviews at [Florida International University], so if you not going to pay me, I'd rather go there." Although I was astonished the first time this occurred, I came to understand it as part of the culture of research in which informants have begun to expect, demand, and receive certain levels of compensation for their valuable time and energy. My anthropological training has taught me that those who need to be compensated often will not provide accurate or truthful narratives. However, I found in my fieldwork that many informants, who have been overwhelmed with requests to participate in research studies, expect compensation for what they feel is a valuable service that they are rendering. These are issues that we as anthropologists must discuss openly and honestly in future debates about methodology and ethics.

When I did gaining entry, I was able to remain welcome only through demonstrating my expertise and offering free labor. One of the first providers that I met with, an HIV/AIDS educator and outreach worker, refused to work with me until I was certified locally in basic HIV/AIDS knowledge and HIV/AIDS testing and counseling. When I told her about my training and prior experience with working in HIV/AIDS research, she stood firm and reasoned that it was important for me to understand what she called "local" problems in the field of HIV/AIDS. So I completed training in HIV/AIDS prevention, testing, and counseling in order to work with particular individuals and institutions, and these certifications helped me gain credibility and legitimacy with providers as an expert in the field of HIV/AIDS prevention. In addition, Haitians who were used to my constant presence at health and social agencies and in the community often assumed that I was HIV-positive, even though I was never asked my status nor did I reveal it. I am unsure how much this assumption helped me sustain long-term relationships with individuals. By negotiating expertise across multiple sites, embarking on additional training, having an unknown HIV status, and offering nonmonetary compensation, I was able to gain entry to and work in multiple field sites. Thus, where appropriate, I include myself in the descriptions of experiences throughout this book. As was true of those who shared their lives and work with me, my identity and positionality mattered, and they affected the relationships and interactions described in this book.

Organization of the Book

I investigated multiple field sites within HIV/AIDS prevention and intervention programs to document how they function and become part of everyday life for many Haitians in Miami. The book is divided into chapters that reflect various

shifts in analyses that continually change and flow to mirror the varying relations between different powerful and not-so-powerful constituents. Each chapter examines the complex entanglements between everyday practices of public
health prevention programming and the broader logics of power operating
across science, governing bodies of HIV/AIDS programs, and society.

Chapter 2, "Treating the Numbers: HIV/AIDS Surveillance, Subjectivity, and
Risk," focuses on numerical subjectivities, or the ways in which we come to
know and govern ourselves through quantification and categories of risk, race,
and ethnicity. I explore the various levels of surveillance that structure HIV/AIDS
prevention programs and highlight the fact that—even though universal notions
of identity and subjectivity become entangled in numerical considerations—
particular groups of people still come to be identified with certain diseases,
such as HIV/AIDS. By examining the deployment and interpretation of HIV/AIDS
statistical data among Haitians in Miami, I illustrate how identities, through
categories such as "heterosexual" and "high-risk groups" circulate, gain traction, and become meaningful for public health institutions and the people they
seek to manage.

Chapter 3, "Treating Culture: The Making of Experts and Communities,"
examines HIV/AIDS prevention experts' increasing shift in focus from individual-
level interventions to those that target whole communities and their cultures. I
contend that this shift has had the effect of making notions of risk, community,
and culture into invariable and essentialized entities and naturalizing the links
between certain categories of people and specific diseases. This focus on communities also obscures the complex ways in which Haitians conceptualize community and culture as sites of both disengagement and belonging.

Chapter 4, "Treating Citizens: The Promise of Positive Living," documents
how positive living—a key component of HIV/AIDS prevention programming
that emphasizes self-sufficiency, medical compliance, and personal empowerment vis-à-vis HIV/AIDS—operates in Miami. I outline how positive living is
linked to broader illness-based identity movements; how it integrates concepts
of self-responsibility with responsibility to various others; how it is characterized by a set of social and behavioral practices that form the foundation of HIV/
AIDS prevention (adherence, disclosure, and safe sex); and how its strategies
are those of "biological citizenship," a set of new dynamic relationships across
biology, rights-based politics, and identity. By outlining the various ways that
positive living functions in Miami, I show how the ideals of positive living are
not always viable or possible for Haitians due to continuing legacies of punitive
economic, immigration, and social policies.

Chapter 5, "Treating the Nation: Health Disparities and the Politics of Difference," explores how programs aimed at specific racial and ethnic groups have
become a normal and natural part of HIV/AIDS prevention efforts in Miami. In

particular, I am interested in why concepts of race and ethnicity are foundational to the understanding of health disparities and how they are entwined
in the discourses and practices of HIV/AIDS prevention in the United States.
In documenting how racial and ethnic differences in HIV/AIDS-related health
outcomes come to be naturalized as common facts that no longer need to be
explained or debated, I illustrate how health disparities have become highly
influential in the science and practice of public health, controlling and generating subjectivities, global policies, and research initiatives. I argue that by
shifting our focus to the generative and productive capacity of health disparities, we may be able to make more progress in improving healthcare access and
outcomes.

Chapter 6, "Treating the West: Afterthoughts on Future Directions," presents my conclusions. In this chapter, I assert that research on HIV/AIDS in non-
Western countries presupposes undifferentiated "Western" medical and public
health paradigms that impose prepackaged views on developing nations. This
is an important analytic tool for understanding the ways in which many marginalized and underserved groups negotiate various medical and public health
interventions. I argue that if we want to move beyond the oppositional dichot-
omies of disease-specific individual and structural interventions, we need to
think seriously about economically, politically, and socially marginalized populations in the United States and how they come to interpret and refute health
interventions and constructions of difference. We need to be innovative and
realistic about possible solutions, ones that involve the cooperation of academics, communities, and policy makers. Most important, we need to understand
that changing the context of peoples' lives for the better is a wholly unsustain-
able venture if the structures and policies, including those of science and public
health, that contributed to the existing inequitable conditions in the first place
are glossed over and left intact.

2

Treating the Numbers

HIV/AIDS Surveillance, Subjectivity, and Risk

On a hot and humid day in Miami, about twenty-five people trickled into a Miami General Hospital classroom for a lecture by Dr. Cruz, an HIV/AIDS specialist. Most members of the audience were African American clients enrolled in HIV/AIDS prevention classes; a few were Kreyòl- and Spanish-speaking clients. Two women led the class in an impromptu discussion of a book on self-education titled *Natural Cures "They" Don't Want You to Know About* (Trudeau 2004), prompting a debate about the validity of the book's claim that drug companies don't want anyone to find a cure because then they wouldn't be able to sell their drugs.[1] The topic sparked a lot of interest, and the room grew noisy with chatter about pharmaceutical companies and antiretroviral drugs. In the middle of this discussion, Dr. Cruz came in. His entrance was like something out of a movie: time and motion seemed to slow down, and the room became abruptly silent as a film set does when the dashing hero enters a scene for the first time. Dr. Cruz was young and boyishly handsome, with shiny black hair that kept getting into his eyes. He smiled to acknowledge some of his patients, and we all watched in awe as he took off his white coat.

Suddenly, as if on cue, Mary Long—a very thin and fragile African American woman who attended these meetings regularly—proclaimed with enthusiasm and pride, "I am 400 CD4 count and 250 viral load.[2] I am the person that I am today because of this man." Her public declaration caught everyone off guard, even Dr. Cruz, who began to blush as Mary showered him with accolades. Perhaps to conceal his embarrassment, Dr. Cruz did not acknowledge her comments directly. Instead he said: "These venues are wonderful in interacting with you because we only get twenty minutes with our patients and that includes administrative tasks." He spoke about virology, adherence to antiretroviral treatment, and doctor-patient relationships. He ended by declaring: "In medical school, our teachers told us that 'half of what we teach will change and the other half might not be true,' so remember that medicine is a trial-and-error game." At the end of the lecture, the audience gave Dr. Cruz a standing ovation as he thanked them for their attendance.

This was not the first time I heard HIV-positive individuals frame and portray themselves through numbers and statistical calculations. For instance, during a 2005 World AIDS Day celebration, Jenisa Mann, an African American guest speaker, introduced herself by reciting a poem titled "Celebration," which narrated her transformation from someone with a viral load of 178,000 and a 33 CD4 count into someone with a "second chance at life." She recounted feeling "dead" when she first learned the significance of her earlier numbers, but through self-motivation and encouragement from social and medical support networks, she made it her goal to "bring the numbers to the right place." Like Jenisa, during HIV/AIDS county-level planning board meetings a white man named "Slim Jim" always introduced himself by his current CD4 count and viral load. He would discuss how his CD4 count had decreased as a result of certain policies enacted by the board despite his objections or express his sense of well-being through his CD4 count and viral load when a policy he favored was passed by the board. Slim Jim was one of the few HIV-positive members on the board, and he used these numbers to embody the negative or positive effects of the board's decisions.

Numerical Subjectivity

Numbers and the ensuing practices of classification and categorization have long been critical in the management of population health because they make evident certain realities on the ground (Foucault 1979; R. Williams 1979). Numerical knowledge of populations has been associated with many modern state-building projects and represents ways through which individuals, groups, and nations are rendered as objects and subjects of scrutiny (Rabinow 1999; Rose 2007). However, it is not the simple presence of numbers that defines public health discourses; rather, it is the burgeoning use of statistics—the science of collecting, analyzing, and interpreting numerical data—that plays a fundamental role in how diseases and populations come to be known and acted on. Statistics are more than social data or techniques used to uncover veiled implications of numbers; they are a language of what I call numerical subjectivity, in which numerical considerations play a critical role in how life is both imagined and lived. Numerical subjectivity allows certain individuals and groups, like Jenisa, Slim Jim, and Mary, to come to know themselves and allows us to recognize them in new and myriad ways. Through cellular statistics and hematological and virological calculations, they (and we) communicate ways of being and belonging, imagining bodies as objects of medical knowledge and numbers as markers of suffering as well as personal triumph and achievement.

In this chapter, I illustrate the growing significance of quantification in HIV/ AIDS prevention, building on other work on enumeration and statistics in the overall management of nation-states and their citizens (Bowker and Star 1999; Briggs and Mantini-Briggs 2003; Fordyce 2008; Foucault 1977, 1978, 1979, 2003; Hacking 1982, 1986; Lorway et al. 2009; Nelson 2009; Porter 1995; Rose 1999; Sangaramoorthy 2012; Sangaramoorthy and Benton 2012; Strathern 2000). My intention is not to deconstruct statistical data, determine their accuracy, or draw attention to faulty methodology or assumptions as shortcomings (Cooper and David 1986; Krieger 1994, 2000a; McMichael 1995). Rather, I am interested in learning how people living with HIV/AIDS come to know themselves and become known politically, socially, and medically through enumeration. To do this, I ask the following questions: How do techniques of enumeration in public health shape and reconfigure numerical subjectivity? Why and how have the categories based on race, ethnicity, and risk become central to discourses of HIV/AIDS prevention? In what ways do individuals and groups come to know the social and epidemiological categories of self and other that result from enumeration?

I explore these questions by tracing the circulation of HIV/AIDS statistics in their multiple forms at various levels: the national HIV/AIDS surveillance reports generated by the Centers for Disease Control and Prevention (CDC), those used by local departments of health (DOHs) in the training of HIV/AIDS prevention experts, and those that permeate the everyday discourses of clients in HIV/AIDS prevention programs. Here, I am interested in how and why certain numbers and categories travel and how particular forms of information and knowledge about HIV/AIDS circulate. I do not take this circulation to be self-evident or assume that meaning about HIV/AIDS is simply transmitted (Briggs 2005; B. Lee and LiPuma 2002; Leshkowich 2007; Tsing 2005). I argue that certain calculations, by their very movement, enable HIV/AIDS statistics and risk categories to be what the sociologist Bruno Latour (1987, 227) calls immutable mobiles, materials meant to flow from one site to another without change. In the field of HIV/AIDS, statistical enumerations of diseased bodies ideally flow "up"—from individuals to local testing sites to city- and state-level DOHs to the CDC and global institutions—while knowledge about HIV/AIDS and resulting categories of risk is supposed to move "down," in the opposite direction.

But, as I will demonstrate in this chapter, controversies about recent transformations in HIV/AIDS surveillance technologies such as the Program Evaluation and Monitoring System (PEMS) and the Serological Testing Algorithm for Recent HIV Seroconversions (STARHS) illustrate that processes meant to standardize data and audit those involved in data collection often have unintended consequences. I also highlight the limitations of existing HIV/AIDS risk transmission categories. I posit that these practices and technologies of enumeration make possible seemingly fluid and self-evident translations of complex structural and social factors into comparable and discrete categories, while simultaneously claiming that these standardized data variables represent real and factual maps of the epidemic.

Technologies of surveillance systems such as PEMS and STARHS are key sites of "friction," what the anthropologist Anna Tsing calls "the awkward, unequal, unstable, and creative qualities of interconnection across difference" (2005, 4). I argue that there is a great deal of friction in the production of knowledge and facts about HIV/AIDS. HIV/AIDS is as much about biomedicine and technology as it is about meanings, definitions, and attributions (Treichler 1999). Technological systems, public health prevention programs, and HIV-positive people routinely engage in messy encounters on multiple scales in linking HIV/AIDS to a series of preexisting worldviews, institutional discourses, material realities, and cultural phenomena. Analyzing the shifting relations between HIV/AIDS science, the practice of HIV/AIDS prevention, and those affected by the disease is integral to understanding these various sites of friction. Both HIV/AIDS prevention programs and the people they seek to serve in Miami are implicitly and explicitly involved in creating and sustaining these sites of friction through the production, silencing, and distortion of numerical discourses about HIV/AIDS.

I describe the work continually being done by enumeration on HIV/AIDS and, in particular, the ways it shapes the local politics of disease and community as well as the broader logics of the paradox of HIV/AIDS prevention. In this chapter, by examining the use and interpretation of HIV/AIDS numerical data in Miami, I attend to how specific identities such as "heterosexual" and "high-risk groups" come to hold significance for public health institutions and the people they seek to manage. I also illustrate the ways in which numerical subjectivity becomes entangled in enumeration and concepts of risk, and how HIV/AIDS experts and their clients are equally implicated in the production and circulation of certain kinds of knowledge about HIV/AIDS and risk. In so doing, I show that enumerative practices both create and are critical to the operationalization of the paradox of HIV/AIDS prevention, privileging collective responsibility and universal risk as central concepts in the fight against HIV/AIDS while demanding an unwavering focus on difference and disparities in HIV/AIDS morbidity and mortality.

Disease Surveillance and Standardization of Data

In 1981, when the first cases of HIV/AIDS became known in California, New York, and Florida, they were reported to the CDC. This marked the beginning of AIDS surveillance, originally conducted to track the progression of opportunistic

infections of unknown cause, roughly two years before the HIV virus was identified (Nakashima and Fleming 2003). As information regarding HIV/AIDS etiology and transmission became available and the public health impact of the
disease became obvious, HIV/AIDS surveillance was conducted routinely nationwide and was funded and managed through cooperative agreements between
the CDC and local and state DOHs (Centers for Disease Control and Prevention 1999). Although the reporting of HIV/AIDS cases by local, state, and territorial jurisdictions to the CDC is strictly voluntary and the rules and regulations
for reporting by each entity vary considerably, the CDC collaborates with the
Association of State and Territorial Health Officers and the Council of State and
Territorial Epidemiologists to establish standards governing accuracy and consistency to minimize variations in reporting (G. Matthews et al. 1994).

As a result, the processes constituting HIV/AIDS surveillance in the United
States are incredibly complex and occur through multiple collaborations at
various levels. The CDC has declared: "Surveillance is the ongoing, systematic collection, analysis, interpretation, and dissemination of data regarding
a health-related event. HIV surveillance collects, analyzes, and disseminates
information about new and existing cases of HIV infection (including AIDS).
The ultimate surveillance goal is a nationwide system that combines information on HIV infection, disease progression, and behaviors and characteristics
of people at high risk" (Centers for Disease Control and Prevention 2013b).
Surveillance—that is, knowing where infections are flaring up and who is being
infected—is positioned as vital for stopping the spread of disease. HIV/AIDS
surveillance practices, in this sense, provoke accounting through the quantification of diseased bodies and accountability by means of scientific necessity
and moral imperative (see also Nelson 2009). Over time, these practices have
evolved into a continuous audit process, tracking disease trends and evaluating
the adequacy of monitoring procedures, including the processes by which various actors check themselves. In describing audit cultures, the anthropologist
Marilyn Strathern writes: "Procedures for assessment have social consequences,
locking up time, personnel, and resources, as well as locking into the moralities
of public management. Yet by themselves audit practices often seem mundane,
inevitable parts of a bureaucratic process. It is when one starts putting together
a larger picture that they take on the contours of a distinct cultural artifact"
(2000, 2). Throughout this chapter, I trace the constantly shifting and often
messy social processes of HIV/AIDS surveillance by which mundane numbers
and categories are transformed into numerical subjectivities—the vital signs of
individual and collective bodies.

Although the CDC portrays surveillance and the resulting statistical calculations as logical and controlled processes, public health surveillance systems involve the complex coordination of various actors, organizations, and

information technology systems (see figure 2.1). In the United States, local healthcare providers in hospitals, clinics, labs, and counseling and testing sites report cases to local and state-level DOHs. DOH personnel then follow up on reported cases for verification and quality assurance purposes by reviewing medical records and corresponding with patients and providers. Data on individuals—patient and provider contact information, patient demographic characteristics (sex, race, ethnicity, and age), testing and diagnosis history, risk exposure to HIV/AIDS, clinical data on HIV/AIDS-related opportunistic infections, and laboratory confirmation results—make up the pieces of information that are collected and entered into information technology systems. This information is then cleaned or deidentified, meaning that patient records and personal identifiers are encoded to ensure confidentiality and aggregated before being sent to the CDC (Nakashima and Fleming 2003). The CDC produces information about trends in the epidemic, which are then transformed into authoritative facts about HIV/AIDS. The continuous circulation of information, including the perpetual acts of aggregating and dividing data, keeps the infrastructure and functioning of HIV/AIDS surveillance fluid.

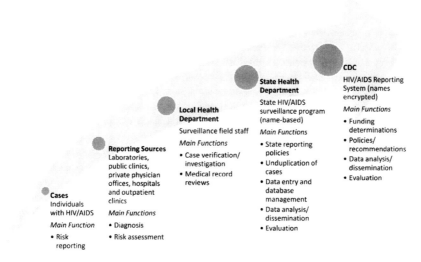

FIGURE 2.1 A flow chart depicting how information on cases of HIV/AIDS moves through the various systems of reporting and surveillance. Adapted from Allyn K. Nakashima and Patricia L. Fleming, "HIV/AIDS Surveillance in the United States, 1981–2001," *Journal of Acquired Immune Deficiency Syndromes* 32, supplement 1 (2003): S68–85. Published by Wolters Kluwer Health.

Changes in Case Definition

The fluidity that characterizes HIV/AIDS surveillance allows for multiple transformations and the continuous evolution of its data collection systems. One
notable site of change has been in the reporting criteria for HIV/AIDS cases over
time, with changes in the definitions of HIV/AIDS cases reflecting the various
ways we have come to understand and define the disease (Centers for Disease
Control and Prevention 1999). For instance, in 1982 the CDC published the first
definition of AIDS: "a disease, at least moderately predictive of a defect in cell-
mediated immunity, occurring in a person with no known cause for dimin-
ished resistance to that disease" (Centers for Disease Control and Prevention
1982, 507). This definition reflected the great uncertainty at the time about the
nature of HIV/AIDS, and only people who had one of the fourteen opportunistic
infections and malignancies without any identified cause of immunosuppres-
sion were classified as having AIDS (see table 2.1).

TABLE 2.1

**Evolution of the Case Definition for Surveillance of HIV and AIDS in
the United States for Adults and Adolescents > Thirteen Years of Age**

Year of CDC publication	Centers for Disease Control and Prevention (CDC) HIV/AIDS Case Definition Changes
1981	Informal case definition established after first cases of Kaposi sarcoma, *Pneumocystis carinii* pneumonia, and other opportunistic infections in immunosuppressed young homosexual men were reported in New York and California
1982	Inclusion of persons with a disease moderately predictive of a defect in cell-mediated immunity and no known cause for diminished resistance to that disease, including those such as *Pneumocystis carinii* pneumonia, Kaposi sarcoma, and other serious opportunistic infections
1985	Inclusion of cases with other opportunistic infections (that is, isosporiasis, bronchial or pulmonary candidiasis, non-Hodgkin's lymphoma of high-grade pathologic type and of B-cell or unknown immunologic phenotype) with a positive serologic or virologic test for the human T-cell lymphotropic virus type III/lymphadenopathy-associated virus (HTLV-III/LAV)
1986	System of classifying patients with serologic evidence of HTLV-III/LAV infection according to clinical expression of disease, including CD4 count and opportunistic infections

(continued)

TABLE 2.1

Evolution of the Case Definition for Surveillance of HIV and AIDS in the United States for Adults and Adolescents > Thirteen Years of Age

(*continued*)

Year of CDC publication	*Centers for Disease Control and Prevention (CDC) HIV/AIDS Case Definition Changes*
1987	Simplification of the case definition to mirror advances in diagnostic practices. Inclusion of HIV encephalopathy, HIV wasting syndrome, and a broader range of AIDS-indicative diseases; inclusion of AIDS patients with presumptively diagnosed indicator diseases; and elimination of cases due to other causes of immunodeficiency
1992	Expansion of definition to include all HIV-infected persons who have less than 200 CD4+ T-lymphocytes/μL, or a CD4+ T-lymphocyte percentage of total lymphocytes of less than 14. Addition of three clinical conditions: pulmonary tuberculosis, recurrent pneumonia, and invasive cervical cancer to AIDS surveillance criteria
1999	Expansion of national surveillance, integrating reporting criteria for HIV infection and AIDS in a single case definition; case definition includes incorporation of new laboratory tests in the laboratory criteria for HIV case reporting including HIV nucleic acid (DNA or RNA) detection tests, HIV p24 antigen, and viral isolation
2008	Case definitions for HIV infection and AIDS are integrated into a single case definition for HIV. Laboratory-confirmed evidence of HIV infection is required to meet the surveillance case definition for HIV infection, including stage 3 HIV infection (AIDS)

Source: Adapted from Allyn K. Nakashima and Patricia L. Fleming, "HIV/AIDS Surveillance in the United States, 1981–2001," *Journal of Acquired Immune Deficiency Syndromes* 32, supplement 1 (2003): S68–85. Published by Wolters Kluwer Health.

The CDC revised HIV/AIDS reporting definitions in 1985, 1987, 1993, 1999, and 2008 in order to incorporate new laboratory testing methods for HIV/AIDS, simplify reporting, improve consistency with clinical practice, and better capture morbidity patterns associated with opportunistic infections (Nakashima and Fleming 2003). In 1985 changes were made to the case definition to include the discovery of HIV and antibody testing, and people with AIDS-related opportunistic diseases could be classified as those having HIV/AIDS if they had an HIV-positive antibody test. In 1987 further changes were made to the definition, corresponding to the transformations in clinical approaches to diagnosing HIV/ AIDS. Physicians were more familiar with HIV/AIDS, and they began diagnosing AIDS-related opportunistic infections presumptively; an increasing number of patients who were diagnosed this way were not eligible to be counted as cases because they didn't have the documentation required under the 1985 definition (Valdiserri et al. 2000). The CDC described these revisions to surveillance, noting: "The term 'AIDS' should refer only to conditions meeting the surveillance definition. This definition is intended only to provide consistent statistical data for public health purposes. Clinicians will not rely on this definition alone to diagnose serious disease caused by HIV infection in individual patients because there may be additional information that would lead to a more accurate diagnosis. . . . The diagnostic criteria accepted by the AIDS surveillance case definition should not be interpreted as the standard of good medical practice" (Centers for Disease Control and Prevention 1987, 7). The changes in 1987 to the case definition broadened parameters to maximize the number of people captured by surveillance. The surveillance case definition did not have to meet the standards for good medical practice; it just had to be good enough to capture as many cases as possible.

The AIDS surveillance case definition was further expanded in 1993 to include those who had CD4 counts of less than 200 or less than 14 percent of total lymphocytes (that is, people who were severely compromised immunologically); three AIDS-defining clinical conditions (pulmonary tuberculosis, recurrent pneumonia, and invasive cervical cancer) were also added to the twenty-three clinical conditions in the AIDS surveillance case definition published in 1987 (Centers for Disease Control and Prevention 1994a). As a result of these changes in surveillance parameters, more individuals came to be counted. In 1993 the greatest rate of increase was among women, African Americans and Hispanics, adolescents, intravenous drug users (IDUs), and people who had been infected through heterosexual contact (Centers for Disease Control and Prevention 1994b). For example, from 1992 to 1993 cases categorized as acquiring HIV/AIDS through heterosexual contact increased by 130 percent. Later reports documenting these numbers emphasized the "spreading" or "emerging" epidemic (Klevens et al. 1999, 80) or the "epidemiological shift" (Hader et al. 2001, 1187) in certain populations. There was little discussion about the effects of the case definition changes in the rise in numbers or the likelihood that these "new" trends made visible by surveillance had been underestimated previously. In addition, by 1993 surveillance case definitions were increasingly employed to determine eligibility for Social Security benefits, and surveillance data were used to allocate resources to areas hardest hit by HIV/AIDS under the Ryan White Comprehensive AIDS Resources Emergency Act—a federally funded program designed to provide a safety net for people with no other resources for HIV/AIDS care and treatment (Valdiserri et al. 2000). In 1999 case definitions were changed again to incorporate newer laboratory tests and to reflect changes in national surveillance, which was beginning to integrate reporting criteria for both HIV and AIDS into a single case definition. In 2008 case definitions for HIV and AIDS were finally integrated into a single case definition, and laboratory confirmation became officially required in order for someone to meet the surveillance case definition for HIV/AIDS.

Changes in the HIV/AIDS case definition over time reveal important aspects of the circulation of numbers and meanings around disease and those who are affected by it. Defining HIV/AIDS is a long, arduous, and imperfect process, highly dependent on the complex synchronization of a variety of actors—including clinicians, epidemiologists, statisticians, researchers, activists, patients, and policy makers. Through the techniques of surveillance, knowledge about HIV/AIDS—what it is and what it is not—has crystallized as unmistakable universal truth, emblematic of what the cultural historian Mary Poovey (1998) calls a modern fact, a mode in which numerical descriptors treated as objective representations of reality involve a presupposed framework of who and what are counted and how to understand the material reality of disease. But as the changing case definitions show, there is much more at stake than just accurately counting infected bodies. These processes bring to light the ongoing struggles over knowledge in clinical and epidemiological work, the connections between numbers and national policies related to material benefits and resource allocation, and the impact of methodological alterations on how particular groups become known or obscured.[3]

Standardization of Case Reporting

Efforts to standardize national HIV/AIDS reporting constitute another important site of friction in the quest to establish knowledge about HIV/AIDS. Reporting practices and policies for HIV/AIDS surveillance have long differed from state to state. Before 1991 HIV/AIDS surveillance was not standardized, and the information collected prior to 1991 is considered incomplete. Since then the CDC has assisted states in conducting HIV/AIDS surveillance through the use of standardized reporting forms and web-based software. Although all fifty states, the District of Columbia, and dependent areas report AIDS cases to the CDC by using a uniform surveillance case definition and case report form, only areas with confidential name-based HIV reporting for at least four years are included in the tabulation and presentation of integrated HIV and AIDS data, so that reporting delays and missing risk-factor information can be statistically adjusted (and therefore minimized) (Green 1998; Hall et al. 2008). All jurisdictions had implemented confidential name-based HIV infection reporting by 2008, and the CDC's 2011 HIV Surveillance Report (Centers for Disease Control and Prevention 2013a) was the first to contain data on HIV and AIDS from all fifty states and six US dependent areas.

During my fieldwork, from 2004 to 2006, data on HIV/AIDS cases and HIV infection were compiled from thirty-three states and five dependent areas that had adopted confidential name-based reporting of HIV/AIDS cases, as recommended by the CDC, for at least four years. Florida is one of the states that adhere to confidential name-based HIV/AIDS reporting, and since 1997 clinics and labs in the state have been reporting positive HIV tests to the Florida DOH (Florida Department of Health 2002). The Florida DOH claims that "approximately 90% of all diagnosed HIV cases and AIDS cases are reported, which is the highest completeness rate of all diseases" (2005a, 3), making HIV/AIDS the most thoroughly reported disease in Florida. In 2004 the CDC began to implement changes to standardize national HIV/AIDS statistics better. PEMS, a web-based national reporting system for collecting and processing standardized HIV prevention data in addition to client and agency variables and evaluation measures, was one technological improvement adopted to bring about this change. The CDC claims that PEMS makes it possible to monitor behavioral outcomes, clients' demographic characteristics, HIV test results, information on notification of clients' partners, clients' use of services, agency indicators, and priority populations, all to allow for the systematic evaluation of HIV/AIDS prevention programs.[4] At the Miami-Dade DOH, PEMS was regarded as evidence that national-level changes did not reflect local realities. Dr. Veracruz, a Miami-Dade DOH official, explained:

> People's behaviors and the impact of prevention are hard to measure. Prevention is prescriptive. Before, the educator had a say in program development. Now, the CDC says, "This is what you're going to do!" The mentality is quality assurance. Staff goes from being trainers to being facilitators. This is a big challenge because one approach can't fit everyone. PEMS is causing a lot of unhappiness and dissatisfaction because it requires us to ask a lot of personal information. The CDC doesn't understand that we do outreach and education in groups and these questions have to be done on an individual basis and it isn't translated.

Many other local officials also felt that quantifying behavior change and program success was complex and difficult, and that certain measurement variables such as number of unprotected sex events or referral outcomes did not adequately reflect the multiple effects of prevention programs. They felt burdened by having to ask more questions of their clients, and in their view the methodologies they were required to use did not reflect the realities on the ground—that is, they weren't suited to the context in which questions had to be asked, and some questions weren't culturally appropriate for certain populations. Many of these officials also believed that their roles were changing with the onset of these new directives. By saying that "staff goes from being trainers to being facilitators," Dr. Veracruz was indicating that providers were being forced to become more accountable to the CDC than to the local public: the top priority of their jobs as prevention providers had become quality assurance, and they were now acting as agents of the CDC to advance national agendas rather than training and educating communities according to their own understandings of local issues. The CDC promotes PEMS as a valuable tool in measuring HIV/AIDS biological and behavioral outcomes and promoting good and efficient practice. But in its standardizing of variables and monitoring of local DOHs and their partnering organizations' performances of a standard set of duties, PEMS is a complex matrix of audit, assessment, and dependency on enumeration techniques and the experts that make them possible.

The restructuring of HIV/AIDS testing forms is another example of changes being implemented in Miami to standardize HIV/AIDS statistical data. In 2006 health workers were informed of a new CDC surveillance system called STARHS. STARHS is considered useful in the detection of population-level incidence of HIV/AIDS; it determines if infections occurred within the past year through the use of new blood specimen testing and additional testing questions. The new questionnaire tries to predict the time of infection by asking clients if any risk factors or sexual relations with high-risk individuals occurred during the previous three months. The most noticeable changes are the inclusion of additional questions relating to risk exposure and the removal of "unknown" categories. For instance, in the older questionnaire, clients were asked if they self-identified as male, female, or unknown, or if they had had sex with a male or female; the counselor marked the responses as yes, no, or unknown. The counselor now asks whether the client self-identifies as male, female, or transgender or has ever or in the previous three months had sex with a male, female, or transgendered person. There are also new questions pertaining to risk exposure to HIV/AIDS, including recent history of incarceration, sex work, and sexually transmitted disease diagnosis (see figures 2.2–2.4).

At Sante Ayisyen, a small community-based clinic in Miami's Little Haiti neighborhood, these questionnaires were introduced in March 2006. Jerome Meus, the lead HIV/AIDS counselor, confided that he was too overworked and underpaid to translate the additional questions without training. For the twelve months or so in which I worked closely with Jerome, there was never a day when he did not look exhausted. Jerome was a large but short man with a shaved head and small wire-rimmed glasses. He had a young child, and to support their family, he and his wife each worked two jobs. They had recently bought a house in Kendall, an area known for its growing middle-class Haitian population, and whenever I visited them in their home, they both showed off their property with eagerness and pride.

I still remember clearly my first meeting with Jerome at Sante Ayisyen. The small building that housed the clinic was haphazardly decorated with items

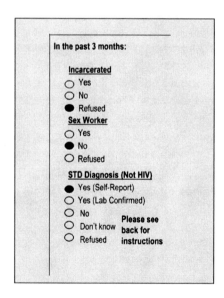

	SITE ADDRESS	SITE NUMBER	LOCAL USE
PERMANENT BARCODE			LAB COPY PLEASE SEE BACK FOR INSTRUCTIONS
	WORKER NUMBER	PRE-TEST COUNSEL DATE	

☐ BLOOD ☐ ORAL ☐ DBS ☐ CD4/8 ☐ V. LOAD ☐ GENOTYPE ☐ GENOTYPE PLUS ☐ RAPID TEST REACTIVE

Last Name   First Name   M.I.
Address   City
State   County   Zip Code   Additional Locating Information
Phone 1
Phone 2   Social Security #   Medicaid #

CONFIDENTIAL HIV TESTS ONLY

Date of Birth	Ethnicity (Select one)	Race (Select one or more)	Self-Reported Gender	Birth Sex	Pregnant	In Prenatal Care
	○ Hispanic or Latino	○ American Indian/ Alaskan Native ○ Native Hawaiian or Other Pacific Islander	○ Male	○ Male		
	○ Not Hispanic or Latino	○ Asian ○ White	○ Female	○ Female	○ Yes	○ Yes
Country of Birth	○ Don't Know	○ Black or African American ○ Don't Know	○ Transgender M to F		○ No	○ No
	○ Refused	○ Refused	○ Transgender F to M		○ Don't Know	○ Don't Know
					○ Refused	○ Refused

FIGURE 2.2 State of Florida Department of Health, Bureau of Laboratory Services, "DH1628 Laboratory Request Form," site-specific information and demographic information, revised in February 2006.

In the past 3 months:

Incarcerated
○ Yes
○ No
● Refused

Sex Worker
○ Yes
● No
○ Refused

STD Diagnosis (Not HIV)
● Yes (Self-Report)
○ Yes (Lab Confirmed)
○ No
○ Don't know   **Please see**
○ Refused   **back for instructions**

FIGURE 2.3 State of Florida Department of Health, Bureau of Laboratory Services, "DH1628 Laboratory Request Form," risk factor information: history of incarceration, sex work, and STD diagnosis, revised in February 2006.

that did not necessarily match, and there was very little room for all the paperwork and supplies that were needed for the staff's daily work. Pictures, posters, plaques, calendars, and paintings hung on the wall in no apparent order. Papers, files, and medical supplies were stacked on old shelves that were buckling under their weight. When I walked into Jerome's office, it too was small, cramped, and in disrepair. The walls were so thin that you could hear the person in the next office. Patients' files were strewn about—along with other

Risk Factors	EVER	Past 3 months	EVER M	F	T	Sexual Relations: (M) Male (F) Female (T) Transgender	Past 3 months M	F	T
Sex (vaginal or anal) with male	O	O	O	O	O	In exchange for drugs/money/other items	O	O	O
Sex (vaginal or anal) with female	O	O	O	O	O	While intoxicated and/or high on drugs or alcohol	O	O	O
Sex (vaginal or anal) with transgender	O	O	O	O	O	With person who is an IDU	O	O	O
Injection drug use	O	O	O	O	O	With person who is HIV positive	O	O	O
Transfusion/transplant recipient	O	O	O	O	O	With person of unknown HIV status	O	O	O
Occupational exposure	O	O	O	O	O	With person who exchanges sex for drugs/money/other items	O	O	O
Sexually assaulted	O	O	O		O	With person who is a known MSM (If client is female)	O		O
Perinatal exposure to HIV	O	O	O	O	O	With anonymous partner	O	O	O
No risk identified	O	O	O	O	O	With person who has transfusions/transplant recipient	O	O	O
Other risk not listed above	O	O	O	O	O	No additional risk or partner information available	O	O	O
Refused	O	O	O	O	O	Refused to report additional risk factors	O	O	O

FIGURE 2.4 State of Florida Department of Health, Bureau of Laboratory Services, "DH1628 Laboratory Request Form," risk factor information and sexual relations information, revised in February 2006.

papers, office supplies, condoms, and testing kits—because there was simply no room for the safekeeping of confidential files and information. To make matters worse, Jerome worked on an older computer, which was always crashing on him as he entered patient information. So when he gave me a weary look in response to my excitement about the rolling out of the new questionnaires, I understood this to mean that he saw them as just another inconvenience added to his already overburdened work life.

Like many of his colleagues at Sante Ayisyen, Jerome filled multiple roles. He did most of the HIV/AIDS counseling and testing, case work, and referrals for clients with HIV/AIDS, as well as street and community-based outreach activities. Jerome's style of counseling was very hands-on. He always engaged with clients on a personal level, asking them about their families and journeys from Haiti. He was much more patient and responsive to clients' questions than some others who also did counseling at Sante Ayisyen.

The first client that Jerome tested with the new questionnaire was an older Haitian woman in her sixties. Jerome explained the testing process and confidentiality measures as he normally did. But as he was filling out standard administrative questions, the woman asked, "If one were to get AIDS, what would happen?" Jerome looked up in surprise and explained HIV/AIDS transmission and the procedures following a HIV-positive result. The older woman nodded quietly, staring off into space. After obtaining her previous testing history, Jerome asked whether she was male, female, or both, and she said, "*Comment?* [What?]" She giggled nervously, but Jerome didn't crack a smile. Instead, he explained dryly, "There are people who change from one sex to another."

She responded quietly, "Female." Jerome often looked confused about what to mark on the questionnaire, and the session took longer to complete than usual because he was translating the new questionnaire into Kreyòl without instructions or training. He then asked if she slept "with men, women, or both," again translating "transgender" as "both." The woman answered "man and woman," meaning that her sexual relationships included a man and a woman. Jerome looked up suddenly and said, "What? You sleep with men and women?" Again, he focused on his own newly created third category of "both." The woman looked confused and then giggled nervously, saying, "No. No. What? I sleep with men only! What kind of question is this?" Perhaps to conceal his own confusion, Jerome ignored her and silently marked "men.'"He then interpreted the question "Are you a sex worker?" as "Are you someone who has sex for money or other things?" The woman responded by saying again, "What? No!" Her reactions suddenly stopped, and she answered the remaining questions without further comment.

The new questionnaire, in the context of this Haitian clinic, exemplifies the difficult translations (literal and otherwise) that are often negotiated between counselors and clients. Jerome was forced to translate into a different language, without any training, the questions designed to accommodate new categories; in the process, he had to deal with different ways of understanding sexuality, gender, and risk categories. The clients he interviewed often seemed confused and, at times, outraged by the survey's recent integration of complex categories of sexuality and identity. Jerome's interaction with the woman, centered on the questionnaire, highlights the ambiguous nature of standardized variables that often do not circulate as they are intended to or that do not produce valid or reliable results that feed back into surveillance statistics. These moves to standardize HIV/AIDS statistical data, through changes to testing questionnaires and technological programs such as PEMS, underscore the complex social processes through which facts about HIV/AIDS are made and remade and highlight the fact that multiple actors (including institutions, providers, and clients) are involved in the practices of this knowledge making.

The Moral Cartography of HIV/AIDS

PEMS and STARHS exemplify what many researchers call "triangulation," the processes of incorporating data from multiple domains to support a particular theory or hypothesis in order to reduce the uncertainty that results from the use of a single data set. The sociologist Janet Shim states that triangulation has "several unintended yet important consequences: obscuring local uncertainties while emphasizing the ultimate 'truth' of a multifaceted model, and minimizing individual differences in favor of generalized, simplified findings" (2002,138).

As illustrated in the examples above, PEMS and STARHS, through triangulation, allow for the obscuring of complex structural factors and social dynamics such as poverty, immigration policy, and racism that contribute to the social context of vulnerability to disease in Miami, translate broader identities such as gender and sexuality into discrete biomedical categories and calculable standardized variables, and represent these processes of standardization and resulting categories as "real" estimates of the epidemic's status.

Triangulation, on a broader level, facilitates the "black-boxing" of the processes that constitute health surveillance systems—that is, vital statistics, disease reporting, routine surveys, and laboratory data—and their outputs, such as schemes for measuring and monitoring disease, guidance for health programs, public policies, and funding priorities. Triangulation allows for the simultaneous erasure and transformation of the multiple interconnecting social and material histories from which HIV/AIDS data emerge. The rendering of these histories as invisible strengthens the potency of HIV/AIDS surveillance and allows resulting data to appear flawless and absolute (Bowker and Star 1999). For instance, compulsory training workshops for HIV/AIDS service providers in Miami start with worldwide, national, and local HIV/AIDS statistics. In one such workshop that I attended, the audience was told that "there are sixty-five million infected worldwide, with thirty-eight million living with AIDS, and new infections happen at the rate of nine per minute, fourteen thousand per day, and five million per year. Half of all new infections are among ages fifteen to twenty-four, and 67 percent of all infections are in sub-Saharan Africa." Here, instructors teach providers to read HIV/AIDS statistics as indicative of the numbers (sixty-five million, thirty-eight million) and the types of people who are infected (those ages fifteen to twenty-four, Africans) and the speed at which these infections occur (per minute, per day, per year). As a result, we come to see the epidemic as an entity unto itself, greater than the sum of its parts, expanding and contracting over time, unconnected to local lives and communities.

We then were shown a series of HIV/AIDS maps, color-coded to indicate either the numbers or concentrations of HIV/AIDS infections. The first was a world map that depicted the number of HIV/AIDS infections by each continent and used darker colors to indicate higher concentrations of the epidemic. The numbers plotted on this map conveyed the spatial extension of HIV/AIDS; the colors seemed to indicate the existence and movement of the epidemic, with a kind of ground zero radiating from sub-Saharan Africa. The second map was of the United States, and the trainer instructed us to look closely at this map. She indicated that each year "forty thousand new infections" occurred in the United States and "10 percent" of those infections occurred in Florida. By showing us the world and country maps sequentially, trainers are asking us implicitly to understand and interpret the epidemic on two different scales: the global level and the local one. We are then easily able to compare the global and local epidemics through the statistics provided. This has two main effects: the revelation of the pronounced gaps and similarities between the so-called global and local levels and the simultaneous distancing and connection between the US and non-US epidemics.

Furthermore, while looking at an HIV/AIDS map of Florida, we were told that "25 percent of new HIV/AIDS infections were in people under twenty-two years of age and half in women." The instructor informed us that these statistics were rising because of "unprotected sex, peer pressure, and a lack of education" and that "HIV/AIDS is the leading cause of death in Florida in African Americans ages twenty-five to forty-four." Through the formulation of scales, the forecasting of future trajectories, and the categorization of people and places (Porter 1995), these statistics prompt providers (and the general public) to infer that numbers are rising because certain kinds of people—like young adults, African Americans, and women—lack adequate education and have unprotected sex. The products of HIV/AIDS surveillance carry moral weight, represent various constituents, and contain invisible and visible mechanisms of categorization (Bowker and Star 1999). The graphs, charts, and maps shown to us in this training allowed us to view the epidemic in multiple dimensions, facilitating moral readings of people and places that these numbers and images represent.

This morass of numbers has the effect of telling a holistic and authoritative story of global and local HIV/AIDS and numerical subjectivity. Such statistical discourses, in the form of maps, reports, and graphs, no longer need to outline their various differing sources. The only connection between them is that they are all related to HIV/AIDS. For instance, the "forty thousand new infections" in the United States may or may not represent part of the "sixty-five million infected" people worldwide. Groupings by age, gender, and race do not need to be presented in the same way or have comparable parameters. What was continually emphasized in the training—"the thing to remember," as one trainer put it—is that a majority of global HIV/AIDS cases are located in sub-Saharan Africa while HIV/AIDS is the leading killer of African Americans in Florida, implying an inherent and racialized relationship between groups of people and disease. Through triangulation, HIV/AIDS surveillance constructs scales that both distance and connect imaginaries of global and local epidemics by compressing and inflating diverse forms of knowledge about HIV/AIDS collected from various sources representing different people and places.

Critical Framings of Risk and Classification

Via standardization, audit, and triangulation, these processes of HIV/AIDS surveillance are foundational in bringing about numerical subjectivity, the way we come to know ourselves and others through numbers, categories, and disease status. Numerical subjectivity is also sustained through the classification structures produced by surveillance practices. The philosopher Ian Hacking (1982) states that an unexpected aspect of enumeration is the way it subversively creates and maintains classificatory labels. Classifications permeate everyday practices and symbolic and material interactions, helping to create the social reality of individuals and collectives (Hacking 1986). For instance, since the beginning of the epidemic, the CDC has been classifying modes of exposure to HIV/AIDS, linking them to behaviors and groups—including Haitians—deemed "high-risk."

Currently, even though an individual can be exposed to multiple risks for HIV/AIDS, surveillance records allow for only a single categorization except for the combined "MSM/IDU" category (MSM is male-to-male sexual contact; IDU is injection drug use). The CDC has employed a hierarchy of these risk factors since 1986 (McDavid and McKenna 2006), with MSM contact at the top, then IDU, MSM and IDU together, heterosexual contact with an individual who has HIV/AIDS or is at high risk for it, and "other/non-identified risk" (NIR) following, in that order. Thus, if a person is noted as an IDU who has heterosexual sex with a HIV-positive partner, the person is classified only as an IDU. As stated previously, due to the changes to the 1993 case surveillance methods and definition of HIV/AIDS, there had been not only a sharp increase in the incidence and prevalence rates of HIV/AIDS, but also a marked rise in numbers of heterosexual and NIR cases (Hammett et al. 1997; Haverkos and Chung 2001).

The numbers within the NIR category are treated as missing data—not as numbers that do not exist, but as numbers that do not fit the model—representing a threat to the validity of enumerative systems by signifying the unknown: the people whose risk cannot be determined and who therefore cannot be accounted for through existing categories of risk. In order to make these numbers count and to erase the uncertainty that their presence creates, ideally the NIR category has to be zeroed out and the numbers moved into more "credible" risk categories. In the 1990s, in response to the growing issue of the NIR category, the CDC developed a statistical method to assign risk factors to NIR cases by using reporting patterns of previously reclassified cases that were reassigned using information obtained from follow-up investigations and chart reviews (K. Harrison et al. 2008). Indeed, during my fieldwork, a majority of cases in the NIR category in Miami were either reassigned to existing risk categories or remained without a risk category after health department surveillance follow-ups, while others were reclassified using a standard reporting delay adjustment weight "according to the distribution appropriate for the sex and race/ethnicity of the case" (Green 1998, 146). Increasingly, the procedures for investigating NIR cases have moved from ascertaining a risk factor for each reported case to estimating risk factor distributions from more "objective" statistical models. With the release of the 2007 volume of the *HIV Surveillance Report*, the CDC began using multiple imputation to assign risk factors to cases that were being reported without them. The CDC stated: "Because a substantial proportion of cases of HIV infection and AIDS are reported to CDC without an identified risk factor, a statistical approach—multiple imputation—has been used in this report to assign a risk factor for these cases. Multiple imputation is a statistical approach in which each missing risk factor is replaced with a set of plausible values that represent the uncertainty about the true, but missing, value" (Centers for Disease Control and Prevention 2009, 60). Multiple imputation allows for the substitution—the filling in—of missing values based on prediction models that are calculated multiple times.[5] Because it replaces missing values with a random set of plausible values instead of a single value, multiple imputation is said to be more objective and automated and produce "less biased" estimates than previous risk redistribution methods (K. Harrison et al. 2008, 626). Accounting for people in the NIR category through increasingly statistically rooted reclassification schemes such as multiple imputation is highly contingent on imported numbers that are random, plausible, and do not necessarily refer back to the processes used to estimate uncertainty—numbers that are there "not to refer to a transaction but simply to rectify the books"—and on achieving the ideal zero balance that, as a result, becomes a "matter of formal precision, not referential accuracy" (Poovey 1998, 54–55).

The Florida DOH reported that as of the end of 2005, the state had higher percentages of heterosexual and NIR cases and lower MSM and IDU cases than the United States as a whole did. In Miami, growing numbers of the high-risk heterosexual and NIR categories were considered a problem by county health surveillance managers, and reassigning cases to other standard high-risk categories like MSM or IDU was deemed a success (Florida Department of Health 2004b). Therefore, in Miami, the directive is to zero out the numbers in the NIR category and reassign these numbers to preexisting risk categories. County health department surveillance managers, when facing high numbers of cases that are categorized as NIR, instruct providers to ascertain risk better, assign NIR coordinators to follow up with NIR cases, and use various statistical methods such as multiple imputation to reassign those cases to more traditional high-risk categories such as MSM or IDU.

A high percentage of Haitians in Florida fall into these problem categories. The redistribution of Haitian NIR cases has resulted in an increase in numbers in the "heterosexual" category. According to the Florida DOH, with the NIR cases redistributed, "the major mode of transmission for cumulative adult HIV/AIDS cases in Haitians was through heterosexual contact (78%) while men who have sex with men accounted for 17% and injecting drug users 4%. Other risks, such as transfusions, hemophilia, and mother with HIV+ status, accounted for 1% of the cases reported in Haitians" (Florida Department of Health 2004a, 1).

During the time of my research, there was some uncertainty as to whether heterosexual sex was an "official" category in the hierarchy used to denote transmission risk. Many patient advocates at this time were calling for the reformulation of risk factors to produce a better understanding of the impact on women and minority populations who often are designated as having "heterosexual" or "non-identified" risk (Espinoza et al. 2007; Hader et al. 2001; Mokotoff et al. 2007; National Women and AIDS Collective 2008). Some asserted that the surveillance system was flawed and argued that the presumed "heterosexual" transmission category only captured people who can report specific heterosexual contact with a partner who has or is at increased risk for HIV infection (for example, a woman who has had heterosexual contact with an IDU or MSM). Often people are not certain about their partners' HIV/AIDS status or risk (Centers for Disease Control and Prevention 1989; National Women and AIDS Collective 2008; W. Smith and Payne 1998). Others argued that the addition of an official heterosexual category would only re-create singular conceptions of risk rather than allowing for a better understanding of how individuals and groups are left vulnerable because of a variety of economic, political, and social factors (Dworkin 2005; Zierler and Krieger 1997).

Despite these growing criticisms, the CDC and numerous public health researchers continued to present the rising rates of NIRs as a problem of "poor risk factor ascertainment" and worked to improve the ascertainment methods through "scientifically designed projects," such as multiple imputation to assign risk factors for these cases (McDavid and McKenna 2006, 289, 291). So it is not surprising that the epistemological ambiguities presented by the NIR category and heterosexual transmission are construed as debates over clinical and epidemiological methodology. Stark deviations from the supposed numerical accuracy of HIV/AIDS surveillance and transmission data in the case of increasing NIRs seem to signify that the problem lies with the collection, analysis, and presentation of information. In other words, officials continue to conceive of the rising numbers of Haitians who fail to fit neatly into existing risk categories as a result of inadequate data collection and disclosure. As a result, they seek to resolve these issues through more efficient surveillance and data redistribution (as in the cases of the NIR and high-risk heterosexual categories mentioned above) rather than by reconceptualizing the methods through which enumeration takes place and the resulting categories that it produces (Centers for Disease Control and Prevention 2001; Dworkin 2005; McDavid and McKenna 2006; Zierler and Krieger 1997).

To acknowledge that many Haitians cannot be identified easily according to categories of preexisting risk factors or that in Florida the major risk factor category cannot be identified for those who test positive for HIV/AIDS (without reassignment to another category) would be to make visible the enormous stakes involved in keeping these statistics decontextualized from the multiple conditions that give rise to them. As the anthropologist Charles Briggs and the physician Clara Mantini-Briggs write, it would be "an invitation to reproduce the conditions that rendered these numbers problematic" (2003, 267). In this way, focusing attention on methods (how to count and classify) avoids having to concentrate on broader questions of the uncertainties of knowledge production (why count and classify) and in the process enables different sets of data to be coordinated without insurmountable barriers (Briggs and Mantini-Briggs 2003; Shim 2002; Star 1989; Star and Griesemer 1989).

The Politics of Numbers

Although those born in Haiti represent the highest percentage of foreign-born blacks living with HIV/AIDS and the second highest percentage of the overall black population living with HIV/AIDS in Florida (Florida Department of Health 2003, 2004a, 2006a), there was no active HIV/AIDS prevention or intervention program that specifically focused on the Haitian population in Florida during the time of my fieldwork, from 2004 to 2006. Officials emphasize that the process of allocating resources to certain groups is complicated but based fundamentally on numerical evidence. Dr. Veracruz, the Miami DOH official, explained: "There are priority groups which are determined by our surveillance department and then the strategic planning committee votes on groups. It's actually a complicated process, where we have all these sheets and we have to check off certain groups based on the evidence." At the time, groups in order of priority for Miami-Dade County were as follows: (1) Hispanic MSM, (2) Hispanic heterosexual women, (3) black heterosexual men and women, and (4) IDUs regardless of race. In addition, out of seven community-based organizations receiving federal funds from the county, three focused on MSM and none focused on heterosexuals. Even though two of the organizations specifically targeted Hispanic MSM (a third targeted HIV-positive MSM), surveillance reports estimate that one in twelve black MSM in Florida is HIV-positive, while one in eighteen Hispanic MSM in Florida is HIV-positive (Florida Department of Health 2006b).

When questioned about the relatively large numbers of Haitians living with HIV/AIDS and the lack of programs for them, Dr. Veracruz implied that the root of the problem was the lack of specificity in population categories in surveillance:

> I think in terms of surveillance data, we need to be more targeted. They classify them as whites, blacks, or Hispanics, but there are many groups under these categories that we don't know if they are being affected. ZIP codes are another way that we determined who is at need. It's not about race but the social environment. We need to further pinpoint high-risk

groups like Haitians or African Americans. We try to implement programs in specific target areas for target groups in areas in need. We still need more, of course. Right now, we don't have anything targeting Haitians.

Dr. Veracruz wavered between emphasizing what the surveillance data do reveal about how and to whom to target resources and what the data do not reveal. Like the surveillance managers told to zero out the NIR category, she argued that further expansion of surveillance methods would be the ideal solution, so that the "social environment," demarcated by ZIP codes, and the broadening of racial and ethnic categories could better tell officials where to target resources for those most in need. At the same time, she emphasized that racial and social environment profiles may not necessarily reflect need. Like many other health officials I worked with, she failed to expand on what and who counts as "evidence" for the allocation of resources and on the complex relations between official numbers and politics grounded in debates over race, disease, and money.

In much the same way, many Haitian community advocates often alternate between using surveillance statistics to point out the enormous need for HIV/AIDS resources in the Haitian community and highlighting how ineffective those same statistics are in garnering them financial and programmatic benefits. For instance, Dr. Charles, who directs a well-known Haitian community organization, told me that it, like other organizations catering to Haitians, had had to reduce HIV/AIDS prevention and support programs over the past few years due to a lack of both public and private funding. When asked about the relationship between resources and surveillance data, he said:

> What happens sometimes is the resources are not distributed the way that they should [be]. Politics definitely has something to do with it. Resources based on surveillance data . . . I don't know about that. You see a lot of resources, for example, in South Beach. Yes, the surveillance data shows that there is a high rate there, but what happens also is that the people from South Beach—most of them are white, gay people who are educated people that put pressure on the system. Yes, you do have resources located, resources applied to African American communities, and that's much better than it was twenty years ago or fifteen years ago. But I don't see that in the Haitian community. I don't really see improvement in terms of services and things like that in the Haitian community per se. You don't have a center in this area, and this is Little Haiti, so they're supposed to have to travel to get the services.
>
> I don't know why that is. Maybe politics, maybe because there is not that many people who advocate for the Haitian community. I still am not satisfied with the level of health resources placed in the Haitian community. That makes accessibility more difficult. So these are the main issues.

By presenting surveillance as evidence of both need and deficiency, these advocates underscore the fact that official conceptions of surveillance data as gospel—as divine and infallible text—is nothing more than political posturing unaccompanied by any substantive action, reflecting broader undercurrents of racial and economic injustices that affect Haitians in Miami.[6]

The Potency of Risk

The categorization of risk in HIV/AIDS—how risk is calculated, who is seen as at risk, and how resources should be spent to reduce risk—as these debates demonstrate, is widespread but contested. Social science scholars have come to understand the concept of risk through three dominant frameworks (Lupton 1999). The first is a cultural symbolic approach, originated by the anthropologist Mary Douglas (Douglas 1966; Douglas and Wildavsky 1982), in which notions of risk circulate through cultural mediums and serve to uphold existing social structures. The second, elaborated by the sociologists Ulrich Beck (1992) and Anthony Giddens (1999), is informed by the concept of "risk society," in which government, science, and industry—institutions integral to the functioning of late modernity—are understood to produce the notions of danger and risk. The final perspective builds on the philosopher Michel Foucault's (1979) notion of governmentality, in which risk is one of the myriad governmental strategies of disciplinary power used to administer populations and individuals, where the emphasis is on the self-management and increasing privatization of risk (Lupton 1999).

Although all three frameworks are important to understanding risk, the third perspective is often used to frame recent shifts in the ways that we conceive of health and illness: from the diagnosis and treatment of illness to the focus on risks and the commodification of health. The sociologist Adele Clarke and her colleagues write: "The focus is no longer on illness, disability, and disease as matters of fate, but on health as a matter of ongoing moral self-transformation. . . . Terms such as 'health maintenance,' 'health promotion,' and 'healthy living' highlight the mandate for work and attention toward attaining and maintaining health" (2003, 172). The gradual move is toward a focus on health and well-being rather than illness and disease, with the maintenance of optimal health constituting an individual and collective responsibility and individuals increasingly becoming—and wanting to be—held accountable for their bodies, health, and well-being (Clarke et al. 2003; Rose 2007; Rose and Novas 2005). Risk is also no longer contained in the confines of the hospital or the asylum; rather, it exists and flourishes in the minutiae of everyday life. It is in this way that we all become implicated as carriers of risk and always already occupy a nebulous space between illness and health (Clarke et al. 2003). Risk ultimately becomes controllable through expert management and self-governance so that to be marked "at risk is to be positioned within a network of factors drawn from the observation of others" (Lupton 1999, 5).

The notion of risk is durable enough to circulate among public health institutions such as the CDC; experts such as researchers, clinicians, and HIV/AIDS counselors; and patients, who are consumers in this case. But it is also ambiguous enough to be the object of diverse and, at times, conflicting meanings. In many ways, risk can be conceptualized as a boundary object (Bowker and Star 1999; Shim 2002; Star and Griesemer 1989). The sociologists Geoffrey Bowker and Susan Leigh Star explain: "Boundary objects are those objects that both inhabit several communities of practice and satisfy the informational requirements of each of them. Boundary objects are thus both plastic enough to adapt to local needs and constraints of the several parties employing them, yet robust enough to maintain a common identity across sites . . . The creation and management of boundary objects is a key process in developing and maintaining coherence across intersecting communities" (1999, 297). Like boundary objects, risk is diffusely and weakly structured in common use, but it has more robust configurations in specific sites such as HIV/AIDS prevention literature, HIV/AIDS counselor trainings, and the daily conversations of Haitian clients. Although notions of risk vary a great deal and mean different things to different people, they have the ability to align themselves across these differences without requiring considerable conceptual or methodological agreement.

Because boundary objects are loosely structured and, therefore, unpredictable and even contradictory, risk as a site of analysis provides a concrete way to study friction between enumeration and the categories it produces. For instance, in a 2006 CDC report on national estimates of risk, the concept of risk is perceived as self-evident. In a discussion of the methodologies used to measure risk, the authors state: "The risk categories used in this report are based on known HIV transmission routes and epidemiologic studies. The behaviors used here to define increased risk are based on the HIV/AIDS Reporting System (HARS), which defines a route of transmission for each case of HIV and AIDS. HARS defines transmission in terms of broad categories (male-to-male sexual contact, injection drug use, heterosexual contact) and not specific acts; the HARS procedure has been followed in this report" (J. Anderson et al. 2006, 4). Without a clear definition of the concept of risk, the authors assume that risk, like transmission, can be categorized.

In addition, they state that behaviors used to define risk are "based on" presumed transmission categories assessed by HARS and previous studies of HIV/AIDS. But the underlying presumption is that the concept of risk stands for behaviors that increase an individual's chances of contracting HIV/AIDS (that is, male-to-male sexual contact, injection drug use, and heterosexual contact). Thus, even though the assumption is that heterosexual contact is a behavior practiced by many and is considered a risk for exposure to HIV/AIDS only in certain circumstances, such as having unprotected sex with multiple concurrent sex partners, the behavior itself becomes indistinguishable from risk. The notion of risk is highly ambiguous. At times, it is behaviors that contribute to increased exposure to HIV/AIDS; at other times, it substitutes for the behaviors themselves; and at still other times, it is conceptualized as something else entirely.

There is also a high level of uncertainty as to whether it is individuals or their behavior that constitutes risk. In the methodology section of the same report, the authors offer a further explanation of the ways in which risk is measured: "In 2003, 45 percent of new cases of HIV and AIDS reported to CDC were to men who had sex with men (MSM), 19 percent to injecting drug users, and 34 percent were accounted for by heterosexual contact. Based on this, injecting drug use and male-to-male sex in the previous year have been used to define respondents as being at increased HIV risk" (J. Anderson et al. 2006, 4). Reportable cases to the CDC are categorized as aggregates, individuals lumped together on the basis of who they are, what they do, or what they have done at some point in their lives. The authors take a category composed of a group of people who have been labeled as MSM; extract the sole behavioral factor (male-to-male sexual contact) that is used to construct the group and, therefore, that defines its existence in the first place; and use that factor to classify those in the group as being at increased risk for HIV/AIDS. Grouping individuals based on one characteristic behavior that leads to transmission risk (male-to-male sexual contact) and moving fluidly between groups of people (MSM) and behaviors (male-to-male sexual contact) in defining risk makes evident the indefinite nature of how risk is conceptualized and used. By being both fluid and situationally grounded, the concept of risk becomes increasingly potent, cultivating notions of numerical subjectivity and functioning in and beyond the domain of HIV/AIDS prevention.

Risk, Race, and Culture

The characteristics of flexibility and invariability serve to naturalize associations between risk, race, ethnicity, and culture that are grounded in official narratives of HIV/AIDS and take root in popular imaginaries. For instance, the CDC states that "race and ethnicity, by themselves, are not risk factors for HIV infection" (Centers for Disease Control and Prevention 2007c, 3) and that blacks also face challenges associated with risk factors for HIV infection, including sexual risk factors, substance abuse, lack of awareness of HIV serostatus, sexually transmitted disease, homophobia and concealment of homosexual behavior, and socioeconomic issues. The official stance, therefore, is that race and ethnicity "by themselves" are not related to HIV/AIDS but serve as proxies for HIV/AIDS risk in combination with social and structural factors such as substance abuse and homophobia. However, surveillance efforts at the national and local level collect and report information only on the racial demographics of HIV/AIDS and not on other social and structural factors mentioned above. Although many health department officials argue that such collection methods aid in the distribution of funds and the implementation of programs to improve health inequities, routine discussions of rates of disease as specific to racial and ethnic groups serve to naturalize connections between groups of people and HIV/AIDS and normalize numerical subjectivity.

Such linkages become firmly rooted through the production and validation of expertise in HIV/AIDS. When asked if there were certain groups that were more or less likely to be susceptible, vulnerable, or at risk for HIV/AIDS, almost all of the providers I spoke to often asserted that everyone is at risk. For instance, Dr. Peters, an official at the Florida DOH, first declared that "HIV/AIDS is about individual behaviors and so anyone can get it" but later stated: "I think that saying certain races are more at risk is purely political. Lifestyle has a lot to do with it. I think African Americans get it because of risk behaviors like drugs and alcohol. They need to satisfy their great desire for addiction and drugs, so they are willing to do whatever. Haitians are housewives who become positive because their men are having sex with different women."

Many other providers simultaneously divorced notions of risk from race and ethnicity while associating behaviors considered as high risk with racial and ethnic groups. Many of them claimed, like the CDC, that risk was not related to race or ethnicity, but to "social environments," "culture," or "predispositions." Equating behaviors or lifestyle choices such as drug use and having multiple sex partners with HIV/AIDS risk while simultaneously placing them in the realm of culture serves to naturalize social and structural inequalities by inherently linking certain groups of people and behavior deemed to result in high risk for HIV/AIDS. In their discussion of the cholera epidemic in the Delta Amacuro region of Venezuela, Briggs and Mantini-Briggs argue that such discourses of characteristics stemming from cultural influences are often indistinguishable from racial and ethnic rationalities of risk:

> When the concept of culture is used to characterize racialized populations, its capacity to essentialize, exoticize, totalize, and dehistoricize is powerfully unleashed, reducing complex social phenomena to timeless sets of premodern traits that purport to provide a self-evident and exhaustive interpretation applicable to all "bearers." Because cultural and overtly racial discourses are both capable of achieving these effects, even invocations of culture that are anti-racist can racialize populations effectively,

and they wield their power without enabling target populations to make
the sorts of appeals to liberal sentiment that would be prompted by overt
public attributions of biological or intellectual inferiority. (2003, 313–14)

Concepts of culture, like those of race and ethnicity, not only function as proxy
risk factors for HIV/AIDS transmission but also implicitly connect ideas of race
and disease to those of numbers and subjectivity. Cultural reasoning allows
issues of risk and prevention to become problematized through characteristics of communities (race, ethnicity, locale, lifestyle, sexuality, and moral or
religious allegiances) and their cultures (standards, rationalities, and commitments) (see Rose 1999, 2007), obscuring the ideological constructions of race
and ethnicity on which they are based.

For many non-Haitians in Miami, articulations of targeted surveillance and
testing based exclusively on biomedical and social categories of race, ethnicity,
and culture serve to connect behavioral risk and high-risk groups and to determine self-management practices of risk such as numerical subjectivity. So when
Karrie Roberts, an African American prevention manager, declared that "it's
just the way it is. Maybe it's due to some biological or cultural predisposition
that we have" in a discussion of why African Americans are disproportionately
affected by HIV/AIDS in a training workshop for providers, no one questioned
or disagreed with her comments. For Dr. Peters, Karrie, and her audience,
not only do African Americans have a natural tendency to be at higher risk
for HIV/AIDS due to a combination of biological or behavioral factors, but this
predisposition itself is immutable ("it's just the way it is"). Here, the relations
between risk, race, and ethnicity have lost what Bowker and Star call their
"anthropological strangeness": "The more naturalized an object becomes, the
more unquestioning the relationship of the community to it; the more invisible
the contingent and historical circumstances of its birth, the more it sinks into
the community's routinely forgotten memory" (1999, 299). As exemplified by
providers' perspectives, the relationships among HIV/AIDS risk, race, ethnicity,
and culture are naturalized and made normal through their grounding in official narratives and popular imaginaries.

Risk and Subjectivity

The kind of flexibility that risk embodies in official statistics is obscured in local
settings, where the notion of risk becomes a dynamic means through which
HIV/AIDS experts construct clients and clients construct themselves as numerical subjects. In Florida DOH training workshops for HIV/AIDS counselors, for
instance, the goal of prevention is "to support individuals in making behavior
changes that will reduce their risk of acquiring or transmitting HIV" (Florida
Department of Health 2005b, II-A-21).[7] Although risk is never defined, counselors

are taught that in order to "influence" clients to "change their behavior," they must induce their clients to "personalize the risk." The training manual states: "A person who has multiple sex partners may not be aware that he/she is at risk of infection because of the common view that primarily homosexual men and injection drug users get HIV. Some who are at risk may even deny that risk. They may not believe information they hear regarding their risk or may ignore it" (Florida Department of Health 2005b, II-A-23). Risk, in both the DOH statement and in general, is treated as an inherent part of the individual, alluding to an internal state of vulnerability.

It is also suggestive of individual exposure to an external danger or hazard. In order to be effective, counselors are told to persuade clients to personalize their risk by helping them take ownership of their risks. They are asked to transform clients' conceptualizations from viewing risk as outside the self (that is, social risk) and outside the purview of one's own actions to recognizing risk as part of the self and under self-control. For example, Jerome Meus, from Sante Ayisyen, asked one of his clients, Lourdes Alain, to take free condoms usually offered at the end of an HIV/AIDS testing session. Lourdes was a large woman who throughout the testing session joked and laughed with me and Jerome as he kept asking her about unsafe sex and condoms. Like many other Haitian clients, Lourdes politely refused the condoms. Jerome persisted:

JEROME: Well, how do you protect yourself from pregnancy?

LOURDES: I've been married for eleven years with my husband. He lives in the Bahamas and visits me monthly here.

JEROME: Well, do you know if he's being faithful?

LOURDES: He has another woman there in the Bahamas. I'm OK with the situation.

JEROME: Do you love yourself more than he loves you?

LOURDES: Yes.

JEROME: You have to take care of yourself. It's important to talk to your husband about protection especially if he is sleeping with this other woman.

With a huge grin on her face, Lourdes told us that her husband was in his fifties, much older than she was, and did not like to use condoms. When Jerome reframed the question and asked her how they prevented pregnancy when he was with her in Miami, Lourdes giggled and replied that they used the "rhythm method," having sex only during the ten days before and after the onset of her menstrual cycle. Jerome kept up his line of inquiry, asking her what would happen if she miscalculated. This only sent Lourdes into a fit of laughter, and she screamed out, "I don't have the appetite for sex." Jerome was not fazed, asking, "What about your husband's appetite?" She laughed loudly and said that he had a big appetite, to which Jerome replied: "Well, then you are going to have to take some vitamins to rev up your appetite too. Only when you eat, do you realize how hungry you are." Lourdes giggled and shook her head up and down to indicate her agreement, saying, "I only realize my appetite for sex only when I am having it."

Although Lourdes was hesitant at first, she eventually warmed up to the idea, taking not only the male condoms but also asking for female condoms that Jerome doesn't offer to clients routinely. In his role as counselor, Jerome was able to alter Lourdes's perception of her risk for HIV/AIDS in this interaction, at least to the point of receiving condoms. By asking her "Do you love yourself more than he loves you?" and telling her "Only when you eat, do you realize how hungry you are," Jerome managed to impress on her that the onus of risk exists as part of her sense of self, rather than as an embodiment of her husband's other relationships or his sexual appetite, and that only she is able to intervene on her own behalf. HIV/AIDS counselors like Jerome are trained to be experts in the mediation of disease-specific risk, transforming individual clients' perceptions of external risk into those of internal risk and obscuring other non-HIV/AIDS threats to well-being.

Clients, as a result, are consistently inundated not only with statistics that relay HIV/AIDS rates of prevalence and incidence, but also with those that represent the categories of who they are through their state of their health or risk of infection. Like many consumers of healthcare, clients are encouraged and expected to get through various prevention programs an understanding of key enumerations (such as CD4 counts and viral load) and risk classifications (such as MSM) so that they are able to achieve numerical subjectivity and manage their own health and well-being. In many ways, statistical data are used "as the necessary foundation for other knowledge" (Treichler 1999, 110), and they underpin ways of understanding self and other in the discourses and practices surrounding HIV/AIDS in Miami.

In clinical and nonclinical settings, however, Haitian clients act to divorce risk from cultural and biological rationalities. One way that Haitians actively negotiate the associations made by HIV/AIDS prevention programs between risk, culture, and biology is by not participating. In Miami, Haitians are scarcely represented in clinical and nonclinical HIV/AIDS prevention programs, compared to other ethnic groups. One of the largest clinical HIV/AIDS prevention programs in Miami, for example, has only two to four regular clients in bimonthly Kreyòl classes, while the English and Spanish classes each have thirty to forty regular clients weekly. Staff members at other clinics also expressed the futility of having prevention programs in Kreyòl because of a lack of attendance. Even the Florida DOH has often canceled HIV/AIDS classes in Haitian Kreyòl for providers because of a lack of participation.

Both Haitian clients and their providers framed the lack of participation as stemming from fear of being associated with HIV/AIDS and an aversion to programs with a sole focus on disease. Dr. Paul, an HIV/AIDS specialist, told me, "When I tell my Haitian patients to come to the Kreyòl classes, they say 'No, I don't want to be mixed up with HIV/AIDS and Haitians.' The Haitians, they don't want to be identified as Haitian and having HIV." Similarly, Johanne St. Pierre, a Haitian woman who had been living with HIV/AIDS for almost a decade, explained, "I'm just too tired of talking about HIV over and over again. I'm not HIV." By rarely participating in programs that target them specifically, many Haitians refrain from associating themselves with HIV/AIDS and avoid embracing numerical subjectivity.

Another way that Haitians act to transform discourses of risk is to claim, as the official rhetoric of universal risk does, that risk is a perpetual state of being, that one is always in a state of risk, and that risk is intimately linked to representations of moral, self-efficacious individuals and is contingent on individual choice. However, unlike official narratives of risk, Haitian clients reject the distinction between personal and social risk and do not divorce the concepts of internal and external risk. For example, Lissette Bennet, a recent immigrant and a first-generation college student who I had befriended through a local Haitian civic group, told me that risk for young Haitians like her was in personal values such as "making money fast" and "low self-esteem." When I asked her to explain, she reasoned: "People who don't want to work—they don't respect their bodies. Instead of working for money, they want fast money easily. But other people have more respect for themselves, their bodies, and they have only one woman. They won't catch AIDS. People right now, they're looking at how to have a good world. They think they need to have good things, so they choose sex because they don't want to work. If everybody works, it [AIDS] would not be easy to catch." For Lissette, "working" is a notion that implies a way of being. She uses the concept of work to imply not using one's body to get material or social benefits and to represent a self-respecting responsible individual. According to Lissette, risk exists as a danger that is simultaneously internal and external to the self and flourishes in the practices of not working hard and in the bodies of those who want to have a wealthy and easy lifestyle.

Similarly Rita Jean, an HIV-positive Haitian woman who counseled other HIV-positive Haitians at Miami General Hospital, was adamant that everyone was at equal risk for HIV/AIDS but stated that "the level is not the same": "I have to do what [hospital administrators] want me to do, but when I am talking to Haitian people I tell them, 'Do not resist what is.' If you are poor, you are poor; if you are short, you are short. We resist so much about who we are and we blame our spouse, our friends, the government, and we don't go to the cause of our problems. We are trying to address symptoms and leave the cause behind. If we want to adjust the symptoms, resolve the cause and then you will have no symptoms." Rita also alludes to the inseparability of internal and external risk, as well as individual and social risk. For her, the level of risk is independent of age, gender, or race; rather, risk is dependent on whether an individual is able to address the "causes" of unhappiness, desire, and necessity that exist both internally, rooted in notions of self-worth and self-awareness, and externally, in the form of substantive and social goods.

Although these discourses align with the official rhetoric that champions notions of a unified response to and universal risk for HIV/AIDS and compels clients to be the mediators of their own risk, they give way to divergent conceptualizations of the self-management of risk. Managing risk, for many Haitians, translates into practices that are not restricted to disease prevention imperatives (that is, practicing safe sex, using only clean needles, and living positively). Haitians who are HIV-positive do not necessarily associate themselves with their condition through numerical subjectivity in the same ways that the non-Haitians in the opening vignette in this chapter do. Instead, many Haitians approach their HIV/AIDS status not through disease-specific enumeration and numerical subjectivity, but through broader representations of risk as part and parcel of everyday life, so that HIV/AIDS is not central to their identity. Veronique Henri, an HIV-positive Haitian woman, declared: "I read books that say HIV causes AIDS and that say HIV doesn't cause AIDS; I get with the doctors, I go alternative ways, change my diet, exercise, read all the books that contradict each other. HIV is the last thing on my mind to think." Sissie Bernard, a friend of Veronique who is also HIV-positive, told me: "My doctor says 'I don't see that you need medication. What did you do?' I say I drank my herb tea every morning. I don't have any problems. That's not a reason for me not to come to see my doctor. I always come to the hospital, I go to all the groups and I learn. . . . I am not thinking that I'm sick; I don't have any problems being sick at all." Both women's interpretations of a HIV-positive status are derived from having multiple choices in the care of the self.

The narratives of Haitians pinpoint sex as the primary way that people are able to get HIV/AIDS, and many reasoned that because of this, everyone was equally vulnerable to infection. Many Haitian women spoke of taking precautions, but these did not always translate to traditional safe sex practices such as condom use. For instance, Claudette, a Haitian woman who owned a tiny convenience store in Little Haiti, brought her husband to get tested for HIV/AIDS at Sante Ayisyen every three to four months. When I asked her why she did this, Claudette reasoned that because she suspected her husband of having sexual relations with other women while she frequently traveled to Haiti, the only way to ensure that she wouldn't contract HIV/AIDS was to threaten her husband with abstinence until he proved via testing that he did not have HIV/AIDS. For her, safe sex could occur and be validated only through testing; it did not consist of using condoms in the face of uncertainty, as is currently taught by HIV/AIDS prevention programs.

These conceptualizations of risk and safeguard practices signal broader contrasts with official norms of risk education and HIV/AIDS prevention. For instance, many Haitians frequently questioned or rebuked the epistemological foundations of HIV/AIDS risk reduction, of ascertaining and ultimately controlling one's personal risk of HIV/AIDS. They stated that one can never truly know about the actions or statuses of intimate partners, and hence official discourses of "being careful" were useless. For instance, Florence Geoffroy, a young Haitian woman who often accompanied her mother on her routine visits to various clinics and hospitals around Miami, opened up to me about how she felt inundated with HIV/AIDS prevention messages as a high-school student in a predominantly Haitian neighborhood. When I asked Florence how she and her friends viewed sex education and HIV/AIDS prevention, she wryly exclaimed: "How can you be careful when you don't know anybody? You can have a husband or wife, and they can give it to you. My dad says all the time, 'You don't know anybody! Don't talk to people!' And I asked him one day, 'Daddy, do you really know everybody? You could never know anybody. I'm your daughter, but you don't know me. You're my dad, but I don't know you. When you go to work, how do I know you go to work, that you're not a criminal when you go outside? How do you know if I don't go and prostitute myself? I don't know you, and you don't know me. We don't know anybody.'"

Florence's comments lay bare the very foundation of HIV/AIDS prevention (as demonstrated in the Florida DOH training manual for HIV/AIDS counselors and by the interaction between Jerome and Lourdes) that one can reduce the risk of HIV/AIDS simply by "knowing." HIV/AIDS prevention is premised on having clients like Lourdes be transformed by what they know (condoms protect you) or by the difficult work they must do in order to know (recognizing risk, personalizing it, and understanding it as controllable) (Foucault 1991). This framing presupposes a relationship between the knower and the known and assumes the transparency of self-knowledge—the ideas that individuals can discover knowledge of personal risk merely through self-reflection and self-recognition because this knowledge is true, real, and waiting to be realized, and that they can also know the sexual and drug-using practices of others. Florence challenges this presupposition by asking "How can you know anybody?" by bringing into focus whether we indisputably know what and who we think we know. She forces a deeper examination of how we have come to see the nature of the relationship between individuals and the rationalities of HIV/AIDS prevention as uncontested and risk reduction strategies as indisputable truths. In the process of doing so, Florence renders visible the multiple obscured forms of social organization, labor, and discourses that produce and veil such modes of knowledge making.

Like many Haitian clients, Florence challenges the very ideas of knowledge production in HIV/AIDS prevention by reframing certain "facts" about HIV/AIDS, risk, community, and subjectivity as socially constructed and as highly dependent on the social relations of knowers themselves (see Shapin and Schaffer 1985). Categories of knowledge, consciousness, and reality related to HIV/AIDS prevention and risk reduction (such as the use of clean needles and the practice of safe sex or abstinence) are not self-evident, but rather are created by the various web of social relationships and interactions that comprise what we know as HIV/AIDS prevention science. In the face of complex historical, political, and economic conditions that render Haitians unequal global citizens, their approaches to HIV/AIDS prevention as outlined here indicates not so much a fierce resistance to biomedical expertise and claims but a detachment of associations among risk, race, culture, and disease naturalized through techniques of enumeration that ground HIV/AIDS prevention science.

Conclusion

Enumerative techniques are central to how we come to know, represent, and act on diseases and populations. HIV/AIDS surveillance and other daily practices of enumeration play a key role in shaping and configuring numerical subjectivity—constructing identities and mediating lived experience. Techniques of enumeration purport to paint a systematic and whole portrait of the global HIV/AIDS epidemic so that its gravity can be seen and a unified response can be coordinated. Instead, surveillance practices segment the epidemic by dividing the people who are affected by it into categories of social difference and behavioral risk and using these categories to guide the collection, analysis, and dissemination of data about particular diseases, groups of people, and the connections between them.

There are many people, like the non-Haitians in the opening vignette, who fervently attach themselves to HIV/AIDS prevention rationalities through numerical subjectivity, positioning themselves as active ethical citizens who formulate and transform their own health destinies. But there are just as many others, like the Haitian clients mentioned above, who conceptualize risk not through numerical subjectivity but as co-constitutive of everyday practices, adamantly refusing to let others—even experts—manage their risk. Haitian clients are acutely aware of notions of risk and individual responsibility, despite expert discourses that circulate notions of Haitians' unsuitability as both statistical data and as ideal subjects and objects of HIV/AIDS prevention. For many Haitians, HIV/AIDS represents a continuing legacy of unequal citizenship, power, and privilege based on notions of racial hygiene and bio-medical and social primitivism. Due to existing biopolitical and public imagi-naries of Haitians as natural carriers of disease (see, for example, Gilbert et al. 2007), many Haitians understand and describe themselves separately from numerical subjectivity.

Continuing transformations in HIV/AIDS surveillance such as PEMS and STARHS illustrate that enumerative practices are highly dynamic phenomena. Techniques of standardization, auditing, and triangulation enable translations of structural and social inequalities into comparable and distinct categories, while claiming that the translations are unambiguous and that their products represent actual and accurate maps of the epidemic. These practices, which work to both unify and fragment, involve institutions like the CDC and DOHs; they also require the participation of clients who are the objects of standardiza-tion. Notions of risk in HIV/AIDS prevention and treatment present productive spaces in which clients are able to exhibit numerical subjectivities, while HIV/AIDS institutions and experts construct them as "risky" subjects. Moreover, as accounts of clinical education programs and counseling sessions demonstrate, perceptions of external risk are transformed into internal risk, and such changes serve to naturalize the associations between risk, race, and ethnicity in official discourses and public imaginaries of HIV/AIDS. Although the transformation of HIV/AIDS risk from social insurance to something that is self-managed contin-ues to occur, formulations of risk are co-constitutive of articulations of targeted surveillance informed by biomedical constructs of race and ethnicity. Haitian clients, however, continually negotiate official and unofficial discourses of HIV/AIDS risk and numerical subjectivities, reject enumerative products to make subjectivities, and refuse expert mediation in the management of risk—in the process, becoming constructed as incompatible subjects and objects of gover-nance through systems of enumeration.

3

Treating Culture

The Making of Experts and Communities

One day in late December, I made my way to the last HIV/AIDS prevention class of the year at Miami General Hospital. Ricardo Garcia, the education coordinator, introduced the keynote speaker, Steve Taylor, as an HIV/AIDS advocate. The first thing that Steve did was to direct the clients, a majority of whom were African American, to move their chairs to make a circle so that they could talk to each other rather than just to him. Then he asked whether there were issues that people wanted to discuss. Arthur Jones, an older man in the advanced stages of AIDS, indicated that he wanted to talk about the side effects of medications, especially the hallucinatory dreams that he had been having while taking Sustiva. Steve began writing these questions down on the blackboard behind him. Other clients, with an air of confidence now that Arthur had broken the silence, yelled out words and phrases like "dementia," "mood swings," and "toxoplasmosis."

Steve was dynamic and confident. With his voice unwaveringly upbeat, he began his discussion by proclaiming loudly that he wanted to "empower" and "self-educate" the participants by telling them about "how HIV worked in the body." Steve then drew a crude diagram of the HIV virus. In response to the drawings, David Roy, a regular attendee of these classes, raised his hand to ask: "How long does an HIV virus live? What is the life span of the virus?" Steve seemed caught off guard and was hesitantly beginning "You know, I'm not a doctor but . . ." when a social worker in the audience spoke up: "It exists for forty-eight hours, but the replication is so fast that there are always more than there are dying." As if not to be outdone, Steve added: "That's what I thought, but I wasn't sure."

He continued in the same upbeat tone with which he had begun the talk. He asked: "What are the cells that are most affected by the HIV virus?" Byron

Miller, another regular client who always sat in the front of the class, answered "CD4 cell," and with a huge grin, Steve thrust his hand into a bowl full of candy and gave some to Byron as a prize for the right answer. Next, he asked the group: "What is the role of the CD4 cell?" People yelled out "fights the virus" and "to protect us." Steve added: "Just remember to think of it as a general in the army that controls how it is going to fight infections." Several people received handfuls of candy for their answers.

Steve went tirelessly on, as if energized by the wave of "correct" answers. He proceeded to draw and describe the HIV life cycle. He explained that the first part was the attachment of the HIV virus to the cell. He asked a question about the name of the entry fusion drug that stops the receptor from attaching to the CD4 cell. Someone from the back yelled out "T20" and "Fuzeon." Arthur, who was growing increasingly animated, waved his very thin hands in the air and inquired: "If it stops the virus right there, why don't they give it to all patients?" Steve again seemed surprised and stood silent for several moments before responding: "I really don't want to get into it right now because I think it's a conversation you should have with your health professional, but my opinion, and it's only my opinion, is that they don't have enough experience with it and in research, many drugs are tested together, but this has not been done with Fuzeon."

Another question was raised by Vera Thompson, who had been quiet all this time. She asked whether HIV/AIDS research had stopped because it seemed as if all antiretroviral drugs were "masking the disease instead of curing it." Steve declared that he would "gear [his answer] more toward facts and not opinions, because there have been many strides made in terms of the kinds of drugs coming into the market. People now can take one pill a day, which is really staggering considering that twenty-five years ago people had to take twenty to thirty pills a day."

All of a sudden, Steve's lecture turned highly technical, and he discussed transcriptases, enzymes, and complex drug combinations rapidly. This seemed to have the effect he wanted; no one asked any questions. However, after about fifteen minutes, James Higgins, a heavy-set man with wire-rimmed glasses, raised his hand and asked: "Do pharmaceuticals share information with each other? Because it seems to me like they should because they could produce better drugs." Steve answered curtly, in an agitated tone: "I think that this is a political discussion, and we can have it after class. When these companies are in the middle of research, they don't share information."

The hour came to an end, and when Steve realized the time, he quickly concluded with the same upbeat tone with which he had started the class: "Remember that you are the driver of your medical care, and everyone else like your case manager and your doctor are just passengers along for the ride. You need to be empowered! Knowledge is power!" The audience responded with deafening applause. As the class was disbanding, I saw him talking briefly with clients, but I never heard him keep his promise to talk to them "off line" about some of the "political" comments that they had made.

The preceding description of a hospital HIV/AIDS prevention class is one in which the production of experts and expertise is highly depoliticized, dynamic, and grounded in practice, and where knowledge about HIV/AIDS circulates in unpredictable and contentious ways. Steve and other experts struggle to indoctrinate clients about the science of virology, immunology, and pharmacology under the pretext of consumer empowerment and advocacy, directly fostering strategies for the regulation and management of health through individual awareness and conduct (Foucault 1979; Rose 2007; Shah 2001). Experts position clients in divisive and oppositional ways, categorizing individuals and groups of people according to whether they do or do not understand modern medical notions of health and illness, conduct themselves in hygienic and responsible ways, and depend on expert mediation for their medical problems. Clients in this class who answer correctly, like Byron, are considered to have successfully understood the science and technology of HIV/AIDS prevention and are subsequently rewarded with candy. Others, like Arthur, Vera, and James, who question or challenge the practices of scientists and pharmaceutical companies are dismissed and their comments deemed "political."

Charles Briggs and Clara Mantini-Briggs have labeled this opposition as one between "sanitary citizens" and "unsanitary subjects." They argue that sanitary citizens are seen as "those who contribute to the body politic by internalizing scientific understandings of health, disciplining their bodies, and sanitizing their environments," while unsanitary subjects are viewed as those who refuse to engage biomedical and epidemiological paradigms about health and well-being, or are incapable of engaging them (2003, 319–20). In Miami many clients in public medical settings, like the Haitians who access Miami General Hospital's HIV/AIDS care, are seen by experts as difficult subjects and uncooperative citizens because of their failure to engage with HIV/AIDS prevention programs. However, Haitians and many other clients who are targeted by HIV/AIDS programs strive to occupy an intermediate state of existence, straddling the realms of productive, responsible citizenship and unmanageable, apathetic subjectivity. Both experts and consumers of health are continually creating and sustaining highly complex understandings and perceptions of prevention science.

I argue that HIV/AIDS prevention experts have become increasingly focused on communities and their cultures as the site of risk and, consequently, targeted interventions. In response to calls to promote health equity by addressing social and structural determinants of health, HIV/AIDS prevention science is continually shifting its priorities from individual-level interventions to those

that target communities. This has necessitated a change in how risk is conceptualized, moving from predominantly biological (race, age, and gender) and
behavioral (heterosexual and homosexual) categories of risk, as discussed in
chapter 2, to discourses of culture as inherently related to risk.

Using ethnographic evidence, I will show that this shift in practice has
diluted notions of community, conflated behavioral and biological traits with
culture, and reformulated the concepts of culture and community as essentialized and fixed entities. This has the effects of naturalizing the categorization
of people by behavioral risk and, in turn, linking particular diseases to social
categories of people. This move in HIV/AIDS prevention toward a community-
level focus also overlooks the complex ways in which Haitians conceptualize
community as a site of both disengagement and belonging.

The Making of Experts

In Miami, like many other places, it is not difficult to locate people who are
commonly labeled and perceived as HIV/AIDS experts. During my fieldwork in
hospitals, local clinics, and community-based organizations, I worked with a
variety of so-called experts, including physicians, nurses, social workers, outreach workers, educational coordinators, counselors, patient advocates, data
managers, technicians, pharmaceutical company representatives, and patient
consumers. Establishing and maintaining credibility, legitimacy, and consensus is a fundamental part of HIV/AIDS prevention and requires a remarkable
amount of work by multiple actors to reconcile the different social worlds in
which they operate (Star and Griesemer 1989). In this way, the construction of
HIV/AIDS prevention expertise occurs institutionally. For instance, local health
departments and organizations in Miami mandate that anyone working in the
field of HIV/AIDS, even as a volunteer, must take at least one on-site basic introductory course on HIV/AIDS science and attend continuing classes, which are
offered in English, Spanish, and Kreyòl. These training courses and workshops
represent obligatory passage points, sites through which anyone wishing to participate in the field of HIV/AIDS prevention in Miami must pass through (Latour
1987). Although I had extensive academic and practical experience in HIV/AIDS
research and prevention, several organizations and informants refused to work
with me until I was certified through these training programs. The programs,
in effect, establish site-specific credibility, maintain the legitimacy of HIV/AIDS
prevention knowledge, and build consensus on how this knowledge is taught
and disseminated (Epstein 1996; Jasanoff et al. 1995; Latour 1987; Shapin 1995;
Star and Griesemer 1989).[1]

I found the trainings to be both substantive and methodological in nature.
All shared an essential thread: the dual positioning of HIV/AIDS, as both a

unique phenomenon and a standard epidemic (Lindenbaum 1998, 2001; Rosenberg 1989, 1992). Trainers singled out HIV/AIDS as an unparalleled epidemic because of specific concerns relating to stigma, as a result of which issues of privacy and confidentiality must remain paramount. But participants were also taught to downplay such unique characteristics of the epidemic to their clients by emphasizing how HIV/AIDS is like any other disease because it can be controlled with medication, leading to a "normal life." Trainees were also instructed to destigmatize HIV testing by encouraging clients to take the test voluntarily.

These training sessions varied from short, four-hour introductory courses to long, multiday workshops for those interested in continuing education credits or certification for specific types of jobs. Given these time restrictions, the classes and workshops were crammed with a mass of information, and their pace was rapid. At the end of each session that I attended, participants—including me—expressed feelings of fatigue and mental saturation. The basic introductory course, for instance, offered participants a crash course in basic immunology, HIV/AIDS transmission, prevention measures, counseling and testing overviews, legal issues, opportunistic infections, treatment strategies, and recent HIV/AIDS statistics. It focused heavily on HIV/AIDS statistics and the distribution of high-risk groups globally, nationally, and locally.

The longer HIV/AIDS testing and counseling training sessions included basic HIV/AIDS information; HIV/AIDS transmission and prevention guidelines; HIV/AIDS prevention counseling, testing, and referral standards; and cultural competency. All of this material was to be mastered within a total of twenty-seven classroom hours, spread over three days. Through a combination of lectures, group discussions, and role-playing, participants were instructed in nonverbal and verbal communication and basic counseling skills that would lead to "ideal" interactions between individual counselors and clients. Trainees were lectured on the importance of transforming counseling session into "conversations" with clients. They were also taught to conceptualize counseling as a process in which "personalized prevention plans" and assessments of HIV/AIDS knowledge and risk could be constructed (Florida Department of Health 2005b, II-A-4).

Counselors in training are indoctrinated in the process of being continually reflexive: they are taught to observe individual clients observe themselves. In the trainings, however, many class objectives went unmet as counselors in training relayed unscripted, more personal opinions. For instance, in a role-playing situation in which participants practiced conducting counseling sessions, one participant (playing the counselor) told another participant (playing the client) that he should no longer have sex because he had just found out that he was HIV-positive. The participant playing the counselor, a social worker, was immediately chastised by the trainers and fellow trainees. In another interactive session, participants were given a list of statements and asked to find other participants who would answer "yes" to the statements. When I answered "yes" to the statement "In my lifetime, I thought I had a sexually transmitted disease," Angel Hernandez, an outreach worker and fellow trainee, stared at me for a few seconds and then said loudly enough for others to hear: "What? And you seem like such a good innocent girl, but I guess you're not!" Nearby participants openly expressed their dismay at her statement.

Similarly, during an activity called the "opinion poll," we were instructed to answer thirteen questions related to sexual health and HIV/AIDS, stating whether we agreed, disagreed, or were undecided. After we finished answering the questions, we were told to show how we had answered by moving to the appropriate side of the room: three walls had a piece of paper taped to them, saying either "agree," "disagree," or "undecided." Statements such as "I feel mandatory HIV testing of all prisoners should be done before their release," "all gays have a lot of sex partners," and "anal intercourse is normal sex" seemed to divide us evenly. In discussions of the last statement, those who agreed with it said that anal intercourse was normal because it was "just another form of sex," while those who disagreed said that it wasn't normal because "sex is between men and women" or commented that they didn't believe that "sex should happen in a spot where you poop or excrete waste" or that it was just "plain gross." Several participants in the class, including three openly gay men, grew uncomfortable as their colleagues spoke of their perceptions of anal sex, gasping or rolling their eyes to indicate their disapproval. Incidences like these were frequent. They made visible the friction and highly porous relationship between what is officially sanctioned as appropriate behavior—illustrated by the standardized behavioral norms made routine through such trainings—and what is considered unsuitable conduct—the expression of individual beliefs and perceptions about HIV/AIDS in professional settings.

The Framing of HIV/AIDS

Experts on the Ground

Private conversations with providers reinforced similar tensions in the framing of HIV/AIDS and risk. First, providers used multiple frames to talk about the meaning of the epidemic (Epstein 1996; Rosenberg 1989). They alternated between seeing HIV/AIDS as like any other disease and perceiving it as an unparalleled epidemic. For instance, Nina Cardin, a case manager at the Haitian clinic Sante Ayisyen, emphasized the powerful symbolic relevance of HIV/AIDS, stating that it was a "window on all those social issues like homelessness and poverty." In the same conversation, she stated: "I look at it like any disease that you just have to control like diabetes, like someone's high blood pressure. Like if you had a headache, wouldn't you go take aspirin, to make it go away and get better? If you were a diabetic, wouldn't you take insulin? If you had cancer, wouldn't you get treatment? So I think of it in the same way." Carole Issac, a Haitian American county health department official commented: "Honestly, I think that it's a reflection of the time that we are living in now. I think that it's like a plague that God put on us for the ways and behaviors of man." Evens Georges, a health administrator working with Haitian migrant workers, confided that he had doubts about the origin and current state of the epidemic. He was well aware that this was a popular conspiracy theory, but he was sure that there was a great deal about HIV/AIDS that we did not know because he could not reconcile existing high levels of innovative scientific advances with the inability to find a cure. He declared: "They are making drugs in HIV research that work miracles, and you can see patients turn around so quickly—and they still can't find a vaccine. You tell me that there isn't something to it. Money has a lot to do with it. The pharmaceuticals and a lot of people are getting rich off of this. There is something going on." These providers, like the counselors in training, are fully vested in the idea of a biomedical cure and are faithful to the scientific endeavor; but they also feel strongly that HIV/AIDS represents individual morality, pharmaceutical greed, and governmental complicity (see Rosenberg 1989).

Second, these multiple ways of framing HIV/AIDS permeate counseling and educational sessions with Haitian clients. As in the opening vignette of the prevention class at Miami General Hospital, presenters ranging from pharmaceutical company representatives and physicians to community activists lectured and led discussions on a variety of topics such as the side effects of drug therapies and the pleasures of sexual intimacy. In one presentation, Nadia Douge, a former social worker and self-described Haitian activist, led a discussion on what she called "the value" of abstinence and monogamy. After a long speech on the significance of social support and open discussions of sexuality, Nadia made those in the Kreyòl class repeatedly declare in unison: "Those with SIDA[2] should not have sex or should have protected sex only in a monogamous relationship." She claimed to be doing this in order to instill the "importance" of abstinence and monogamy. When Richard Jaubert, an older Haitian man with advanced AIDS, became inspired by our chanting and exclaimed in an unexpected outburst that he had not had sex in the eight years since he had been HIV-positive, Nadia led us in giving him a standing ovation. Like the HIV/AIDS workshops for counselors in training, this presenter transitioned effortlessly between established narratives of HIV/AIDS prevention of safer sex behaviors and her own moral convictions about abstinence and monogamy.

HIV/AIDS pre- and post-test counseling sessions were brief, unlike prevention education classes, and the intake form was the mainstay of the interaction between counselor and client and, therefore, the entire counseling session. Frequently, the session seemed like a lecture, with the counselor imparting information about HIV/AIDS virology, transmission, and risk rather than using questions or so-called polite imperatives to encourage clients to explain their concerns, as is commonly taught in training workshops. A few clients asked questions, raised concerns about the relayed information, and divulged complex personal situations; a majority, however, remained silent and answered only the questions asked from the intake form.

Counselors often breached the Florida Department of Health's HIV/AIDS prevention counseling standards by imposing their own opinions on clients. For instance, in a counseling session between Jerome Meus, the lead Haitian HIV/AIDS counselor at Sante Ayisyen, and Lyne Clement, a young Haitian woman who was there to get her test result, Jerome kept questioning the validity of Lyne's commitment to using condoms. He became agitated when she kept refusing his offers of condoms. He asked her sternly if she was responsible for obtaining protection, and she replied that her partner "brought the protection." Jerome then raised his voice as if he was scolding a child: "Well, what if he doesn't come with condoms one time? What will you do?" "Well, we are always careful," said Lyne, shrugging her shoulders. Jerome persisted: "You can't rely on that. I am going to give you condoms." When she quietly refused again, he yelled: "You're seventeen and you shouldn't be having sex anyway. I know you don't want them, but I am going to send you home with some condoms." She let out a loud sigh, reluctantly took them, and put them into her bright pink Hello Kitty book bag. Lyne's assurances of "always" being careful and using condoms did not deter Jerome from insisting that she take the condoms he offered. His invocations of self-empowerment only heightened her refusals until the very end, when the prescribed roles between counselor and client were ruptured by Jerome's admonishing Lyne for having sexual relations at her young age.

Similarly, David Pierre-Louis, a Haitian counselor at another clinic in Little Haiti, administered the test on me in order to demonstrate the use of OraSure, a diagnostic rapid HIV test approved for oral use, and to show me how "real-life" counseling sessions unfolded. During the pre-test counseling session, he checked me off as African American and then, laughing, apologized and said that he was so used to marking everyone black or African American that he didn't think to mark me as anything different. David rapidly asked questions related to my sexual behaviors and those of my sexual partners while he filled out the risk transmission section. He was speaking and writing so fast that his pen often marked the "no" box before I even answered. In the middle of the session, David declared flirtatiously, "I knew you looked like you didn't have too many [risk factors]." I was taken aback by his comments that linked my physical appearance to my disease risk. Although it was a practice session, I was being tested for HIV/AIDS and, in the role of a client, felt highly uncomfortable discussing my sexual history and drug use, or answering any questions because of David's overt judgments of me.

Even though many of the counseling sessions that I witnessed were conducted with professionalism and empathy, they still made apparent the ambiguous and inadequate nature of concepts that form the mainstay of the doctrines of HIV/AIDS counseling and prevention, such as confidentiality and neutrality, when put into practice. Stacey Leigh Pigg (2001) states that contemporary models of HIV/AIDS education have erased the culturally specific historical formation of the modern notion of sex, one that transferred sex from a personal and emotional realm of public discourse to one of scientific rationality. She posits that this medicalization of sexuality made it possible to discuss sex education and safe sex with clinical objectivity in HIV/AIDS programs. I would add here that there has also been a medicalization, and subsequent depoliticization, of the social relations between HIV/AIDS counselors and clients. Neutrality and nonjudgmental behavior are seen as the ideal standards in HIV/AIDS educational and counseling interactions in mock and actual counseling sessions and educational classes. The training of HIV/AIDS experts—in this case, counselors specifically—is based on scientific rationality and obscures the cultural histories of individuals, social relations, and HIV/AIDS prevention. Experts are caught in a bind, vacillating between what is taught to them through institutional training and their personal conceptualizations of morality, sexuality, and risk. Counselors and providers—in the process of dynamically negotiating their position as people who have enlisted in the official discourses of cultural reasoning and who are embedded in the same kinds of moral and social norms that they seek to act on—construct their clients in similar ways, as either responsible citizens or as unmanageable subjects.

Experts from Below

Haitians also contribute to the production and maintenance of conceptions of HIV/AIDS, risk, and community and, in the process, cautiously navigate the terrain between responsible citizenship and unmanageable subjects in the field of HIV/AIDS prevention. Haitians in Miami have a long history of being targeted by local and national HIV/AIDS prevention and research programs, and almost all of my informants and their friends and families had in some way interfaced with these programs through HIV/AIDS counseling, street outreach, or in formal and informal classes in local organizations and clinical settings.

Very few of my informants ever used the words "virus" and "chronic disease" in describing HIV/AIDS. Instead, the vast majority of them conceptualized HIV/AIDS as something that is shared between two individuals through sex or drugs, or spoke about how they would react to it if they had it. Others questioned what they had been taught about HIV/AIDS: Was it really spread through needles or sex? Were vaccines not being found intentionally, because corporations and individuals were making too much money from the "business" of HIV/AIDS? Some offered explanations that merged biomedical notions of HIV/AIDS with their own personal interpretations. For instance, Claudette, the owner of a small convenience store who brought her husband to get tested for HIV/AIDS every three to four months at Sante Ayisyen because of her suspicions of his infidelity during her frequent trips to Haiti, reflected: "I remember one time they tell you SIDA is a virus. Everybody has it in their blood, but sometimes it's not developed and for some people, if you don't do it, it doesn't bother you. If you do prostitution, you can develop more. If you are on drugs, too." Claudette constructs SIDA as a virus, following what she has learned from the medical staff at the clinic, but she interprets this virus to be endemic to the human body. If someone were to "do prostitution" or be "on drugs," then this virus will develop; if "you don't do it," then it will not develop. For her, like many of my informants, SIDA was a confluence of biological entities, experiences, ways of being, and consequences of certain behaviors and actions.

For others, health was inextricably linked to monetary wealth, and HIV/AIDS was seen as a means of garnering resources that were otherwise not available. Caniela Lucas, a divorced mother of two who was suffering from complications related to an overactive thyroid, had spent almost all of her money on medication and healthcare bills. She told me matter-of-factly:

> When I go to Miami [General Hospital], I have no problem to see the doctor. You know that you have to pay, you have to pay something. If you do the papers good, they will give you discount. When I go there, I have to pay $81 to see the doctor and I have to pay all my medications the same. If I bring them all those papers, they will give me discount and I will pay half on that medication. I will pay . . . I think $30 for the doctor and I will pay what my medication will cost. I will pay half or three quarters . . . whatever I deserve because if you miss one paper, they're not going to give you the discount. You have to bring all what they ask you. One time I went to see my doctor and I don't have $81 to see my doctor. I don't have the papers to get discount. I tell her I can't see you because I need $81. Nothing I can do. Nothing she can do for me. That day, I almost died because I don't have $81. The poor are dying. When you don't have money, you die.

Caniela had been working but had had to stop recently because of her poor health. She was so strapped for money that two weeks before my visit, she had sent her children to live with their father because she could no longer afford to take care of them. As I sat with her in her small apartment, I noticed that she had very little furniture: the living room was empty except for three large boxes stacked in one corner, a laundry basket filled with clothes, and some detergent sitting next to it. There was only one small framed picture on the wall, a studio portrait of Caniela posing regally in a two-piece ivory gown with lots of makeup and her lustrous black hair pulled back in a bun. I was startled by how different she looked now—a hollowed-out version of her former self. She had bags under her eyes and looked really tired, as if she had not slept in a few days. She had lost a significant amount of weight, and her hair, eyes, and skin looked very dull.

When I asked her how she was, she complained of being constantly tired and broke and feeling that she had lost control over her life. "My health is not good because I have a thyroid," Caniela told me. "That thyroid give me a lot of complications. It give me heart problems and I don't breathe too good. Sometimes my heart hurt me a lot. I have a lot of problems. Sometimes, I can't sleep because it's not too good. The sickness I have . . . the stress give you that. I can tell you I have a lot of stress because I'm not working, I have two children and I have to leave them and I cannot do nothing. I was sick all the time, sick all the time, sick all the time. You know it's very hard. And my medication . . . I can't buy my medication. I was sick all December because I don't take my medication because I don't have money to buy it." When I asked her if anyone was helping her, she began to cry. "When he [her ex-husband] see that I get sick, he don't help me," she told me between sobs. "I don't know what to do and I tell him to keep the children for me until I get a job and help my children and keep them. But that time, he don't give me nothing for the children. I tell my social worker when he don't give me nothing and after that, she tell me I have to bring this paper, I have to bring that paper, I have to bring this light bill. I don't live with him; he's not going to give me his light bill to go get help. No Haitian man going to do that. [The social workers] don't understand what I see."

Caniela spoke eloquently for a long time about her protracted struggles with health problems, poverty, and lack of insurance. She also voiced her difficulties in obtaining federal and state assistance for economic and medical needs and the various kinds of denials she faced because she did not have access to the necessary "evidence" to prove need. When our conversation turned toward HIV/AIDS, Caniela revealed that many Haitians, including her ex-husband, assumed that she had HIV/AIDS because of her sudden change in appearance. She explained: "Haitians . . . if you lost weight, they say 'oh.' Like people scared of me especially when I lost weight, I lost weight nonstop. You see my husband . . . I leave him, and he go to Haiti and he tell my son, 'Oh your mother has AIDS! Your mother is finished; she almost die and you're not going to see your mother no more!'" She started to cry, saying: "And he say that . . . and Haitians, even here and even in Haiti, if you sick and you lose weight, they say you have AIDS. My husband—my ex-husband go and tell my son, and my son call and tell me 'Mom! Dad tell me you sick.' You know he don't want to tell me the way that man tell him. He said, 'He tell me you sick, and I'm not going to see you no more. You going to die.' I said it's not true, because if I go to the doctor, I'm not going to die. I say I don't have AIDS, and even if he say I have AIDS, don't pay him no mind." She suddenly paused, thinking. Looking past me, at the empty white wall opposite her, Caniela murmured in an exasperated tone: "Sometimes, maybe if God give me AIDS, I can say that it would be better for me. I don't have a house to stay [in], I don't have nothing for my two kids because [the government] doesn't give me nothing. I say, 'If I have AIDS, they will give me house to stay [in], they will give me money.' I have a lady who is my ex-husband's friend. Friends say, 'She have AIDS.' Now, this woman has everything. She has nutrition, money for a house. She has everything. She has money, and they pay her light bill and they give her food stamps. They give her everything. That's why I say maybe if I have AIDS, they will give me everything too."

This narrative indicates the potential value of HIV/AIDS. For Caniela, HIV/AIDS symbolizes a collection of resources that seem easily obtainable by people with the disease—unlike her thyroid disease, which requires her to produce mounds of paperwork to prove her economic and medical needs. She perceives HIV/AIDS as a disease that would allow her to live without suffering and give her access to resources such as adequate insurance coverage, free medications, affordable housing, money, and food. She suggests that her physical and social suffering are similar to those of people who live with HIV/AIDS, but that her suffering is wasted because thyroid disease gets her very little material support. Like her friends, Caniela does not know for certain that her ex-husband's friend has HIV/AIDS; rather, she assumes this woman has HIV/AIDS because she is in a better social and financial situation. In the social worlds of Caniela and her friends, HIV/AIDS becomes the only way that this woman, much like any other poor Haitian, could receive monetary and social recognition. HIV/AIDS, for Caniela, represents luck, prosperity, and desire rather than discrimination and shame, a notion that experts believe helps explain why clients aren't engaged in prevention programming.

The Framing of Risk and Culture

Expert Mediators

The ways in which the notion of risk circulates between providers and clients is crucial to the understanding of how expertise is negotiated across multiple sites. The notion of risk is a core element of the principles of HIV/AIDS prevention and intervention and of the production of expertise in this field. In training workshops for providers, instructors discussed risk extensively, and in testing and counseling practice sessions, instructors reinforced the ultimate goal of the counselor: to extract information for risk assessment at the individual and group levels. However, the concept of risk itself was never defined. Instructors addressed HIV/AIDS transmission routes, individual behaviors that promoted increased transmission rates, and groups of people who are considered more vulnerable to HIV/AIDS, all under the rubric of risk. Conversations and lectures moved fluidly between notions of "risk group(ing)s," "risk or risky behavior," and being "at risk" without much differentiation, while the notion that "we all have AIDS" was a popular quote used to underscore the universality of risk.

In conversations, interviews, and interactions with clients, both providers and providers in training used the multiple and overlapping readings of risk that form the mainstay of the paradox of HIV/AIDS prevention. Many reiterated that everyone is at risk, while also insisting that certain groups of people are more at risk than others. Providers who worked with Haitian clients expressed the view that "culture" or the "nature of the Haitian people" put them at risk, while simultaneously portraying the community as one that was "suffering." Almost all providers rejected the notion that risk was a direct result of being part of a specific ethnic or racial grouping; rather, they interpreted risk as attributable to "predispositions" or "cultural factors" such as "low education and beliefs" that led to risky behavior. For instance, Tony Robles, a Hispanic community health worker, indicated that it was important to pay attention to "culture" and tensions between "tradition and assimilation" when working with Haitians. Tony reasoned that "cultural tendencies"—such as the reluctance to discuss HIV/AIDS, due to the long-standing stigma of being labeled as unclean disease carriers, and dependence on voodoo—didn't really make it possible for Haitians to adhere to new medical recommendations.

Similarly, several providers explained that Haitians were at high risk for HIV/AIDS because their "culture" led to a lack of access to preventive medical care and the incapacity to understand modern medical interventions. Two prominent HIV/AIDS specialists said:

> [Haitians] don't access healthcare because in the Haitian culture, they think that you go to [the] doctor when you're sick. If you are not sick, you shouldn't go to the doctor. Now, they were feeling perfectly well before they started going to the doctor, and when I give the medicine and they get sick because of the side effects, and they think it's because of the medicine. We educate people and give them certain information about the pathogenesis of HIV and the transmission of the virus. We tell them that taking the medicine will make you feel sick because the virus is dying, so therefore it's worth it for them to take the medicine, and the side effects will slowly go away. So you either convince them and they buy it, or you lose them completely and it's a big problem. They also have this thing about the voodoo. In fact I had a couple of patients who have said that "I don't have to use a condom. I am cursed by an *oungan* [voodoo priest]

but my wife is not. There's no way that she's going to get it because I can protect her with my voodoo. Condoms are not necessary." I mean he really believed it. So we had to send him for therapy and use an *oungan* to educate and educate and educate to convince him. (Dr. Bristol)

One reason that I started the Haitian clinic was that these people are very poorly treated, and in fact once somebody said that it was impossible to treat [them] . . . that it was almost like practicing veterinary medicine. The reason that he said that was whatever you say they don't understand, and whatever they say you don't understand. The Haitian people are very subdued. They are not very vocal, so if they don't understand something they may not say, "Look Doc, I don't understand." Even if a Kreyòl-speaking person explains it, they may just keep quiet. And they misunderstand instructions [a] little bit more than others. Like when the pharmacies make mistakes, even if they know, they don't challenge the authorities very much. They are very secretive. They don't want people to know. The Haitians, they don't want to mix with Haitians so that each other will know that they have HIV. And other thing is poverty. Most of them are unemployed. A fair amount are illegal [immigrants], and some of them don't know how to access services. (Dr. Paul)

These two doctors, like many other providers, subscribe to notions that Haitians are incapable of achieving adequate comprehension and compatibility with providers in clinical encounters. They position Haitians as a group that is subject to great "suffering" and use the rubric of "culture"—a catchall term including lack of education and time, low health literacy, immigration status, language barriers, and poverty—to explain Haitians' risk for HIV/AIDS. Some of these risk factors can be mediated through education or "buy ins" because culture can be repackaged as complementary or an appendage to science (for example, using *oungans* to "educate" patients about safe sex); the vast majority of risk for Haitians, however, is deemed incommensurable to HIV/AIDS prevention, implying that Haitians are somehow "naturally" unsuited for common medical interventions and technologies. In addition, historical injustices, structural impediments to healthcare access, and alternate modes of understanding disease and health are all subsumed under "culture" and, subsequently, become naturalized as risk factors.

Alternative Perspectives

The notion of risk frequently elicited narratives from Haitians about lack of insurance, money, and other resources, as well as struggles with bureaucracy, poverty, and family. Many Haitian clients spoke of not seeking healthcare early or often enough because of its prohibitive cost, the rude or unfair treatment they received, their fear of seeing or being seen by other Haitians, and their lack of time. Some complained that although they wanted to get necessary or preventive health services, they could not afford to because doing so often involved taking time off—frequently an entire day—from their hectic work schedules and jobs that did not offer paid sick leave. Nadege Duhem—who worked seven days a week as a cleaning lady, putting in sixty hours a week—told me: "When I come [to the clinic], my [blood] pressure goes up, my sugar goes up. I don't really want to come here. Sometimes, when I come, I feel more sick with these people at the desk. They're very rude; they don't know how to talk to people. I came here at 10:15 A.M., and it's now noon. When you come and spend five hours, it doesn't make sense." Like Nadege, many Haitians repeatedly mentioned that they avoided seeking or were unable to seek medical care because they could not afford to spend time away from work. Instead, they embarked on complex ways of accessing care, often going from one institution to another to avoid accumulating enough bills to trigger a call from a collection agency, avoiding certain clinics and hospitals because of a lack of money or dissatisfaction with rude personnel, or even bypassing medical institutions in Miami altogether to get services and treatments in Haiti instead.

Many clients also confided that they feared coming to the clinic or hospital because their immigration status might result in their being reported to immigration services. There were several times during my fieldwork when many clients stayed away from public institutions, including medical ones, due to fear of potential immigration raids. They recounted stories about "INS trucks picking up people" and being criminalized "for associating with anyone illegal." From 2005 to 2006, there were many intermittent but prolonged scares in the aftermath of discourses in the national media against illegal immigration. Many community advocates worried that Haitians were not accessing health services, and that the situation was reaching dangerous levels. These leaders were aggravated by government officials' lack of transparency in this enforcement process and were equally frustrated with their inability to reach the Haitians who were not accessing services.

Haitians frequently pointed to stigma as a critical reason for their not seeking HIV/AIDS testing and preventive services. Richard Jaubert, a regular in the Kreyòl education classes, told me he thought that many Haitians did not come to these classes because "stigma" prevented them from doing so. When I asked him for clarification, Richard said that stigma signified fear of judgment if their condition were revealed. Magda Renaud echoed Richard's sentiments: "If I tell another Haitian, they will tell others, so I don't tell anyone that I'm sick." Thus, stigma was related to disclosure of personal information and operated as a set of perceived obstacles that prevented interactions with healthcare systems.

A few Haitian clients, particularly those working as patient advocates, used the notion what is often labeled "HIV fatigue" to express their thoughts about why other Haitians were reluctant to attend HIV/AIDS prevention programs. In HIV-positive adults, fatigue is a common but serious and debilitating symptom of either the disease or a side effect of HIV/AIDS medications. It is experienced as extreme tiredness that is not made better by rest, and its impact can have long-lasting physical, emotional, and social effects. HIV/AIDS-related fatigue can be controlled by medical treatments and lifestyle changes such as better nutrition and more frequent exercise.

Clients and providers in Miami, however, discussed "HIV fatigue" as a saturation point that clients reached as a consequence of being inundated with repetitive HIV/AIDS information; it resulted in outright or indirect refusals to engage in HIV/AIDS prevention programs. For instance, a program administrator explained: "The community is become complacent about HIV. Maybe they've become HIV fatigued. They don't want to hear about it. To me, that can make someone less likely to hear the message of HIV." For providers, the notion of fatigue was often associated with indifference and lack of concern, sentiments that would inevitably lead to unsafe practices and an increase in HIV/AIDS in the community. For clients, HIV fatigue was a way to express their dissatisfaction and disillusionment with the structure of prevention programs, which were limited to educational classes or counseling sessions. Magda Blais, a petite Haitian woman who had been abandoned by her family after her positive HIV diagnosis, emphatically said: "It's too overwhelming because you deal with the disease every day, and the last thing you want to do is talk about it more." HIV fatigue for her was not a result of complacency or indifference; rather, discussions of HIV/AIDS had become too consuming and too definitive of her daily life.

Haitian clients openly expressed their desire for prevention programming formats that were less "educational" and more about "support." In the hospital prevention classes conducted in Kreyòl, Haitian attendees often asserted themselves in discussing personal issues. Irene Dorval, for instance, was a young Haitian, HIV-positive, single mother with an HIV-positive daughter. She was different from others in the class: her outfits were flashy and skintight, always revealing her ample bosom; she had a mouth full of gold teeth; she flirted overtly with men in the class; and she was very open about her sexual relationships and her displeasure with not getting enough resources to support herself and her daughter. I often saw other women in the class turn their heads away when Irene strutted into class in a revealing outfit or heard them gossip about her sexuality. In one class, Irene seemed visibly upset, with her eyes and cheeks swollen as if she'd been crying heavily. When Mona Blanc, the Haitian patient advocate, asked her what was wrong, Irene replied: "I have a problem with my daughter." I'd met her daughter while attending a special group for HIV-positive children at Miami General; she was about ten or eleven years old. My heart sank as I contemplated the thought that something had made her sick. Irene continued: "In the class my daughter goes to, they tell the children to share their status with people they are close to." There were immediate gasps of disbelief from the men and women in the class. Holding back tears, Irene continued: "So my daughter told her best friend, told her that she has HIV. This girl's mother come to me and is cursing and screaming. She Haitian. She tell me that she's going to tell everybody. She tell me that I'm putting her daughter in danger. She tell me that she is going to take action against me for not telling her." Irene told us that she was very upset and didn't know what to do. Mona calmly asked: "Is your daughter's best friend treating her any different?" "No," answered Irene. "She be hugging and kissing her. I don't see nothing different." Mona, along with other women, advised her to talk to the best friend's mother: "Talk to her calmly about the disease. Tell her about precautions. Educate her about the disease. She doesn't know and you need to educate her. She needs to feel comfortable and you need to give her time to get used to things." Richard, chimed in: "Protect your daughter too by talking with her. You don't want her to feel bad if her friend don't want to be her friend."

Irene then said: "I'm having some other problems too. I have a lawyer who is trying to get me [legal immigrant] status. He take $250 from me and then tell me that he can't do nothing for me because of some law. He tell me that he need another $2,000 to finish his job." People in the class sprang into action. They told Irene that there were lots of lawyers who did work for Haitians for free and gave her some names to contact. They said that there were agencies that could help her with such matters, and that she wouldn't have to pay for their services.

Almost all participants were engaged and talking in classes like these, where Haitian clients were able to talk explicitly about issues of importance to them—not only about HIV/AIDS and health, but also about immigration, poverty, housing, politics, transportation, depression, isolation, religion, family, and resocialization after an HIV-positive diagnosis. Standard lectures about HIV/AIDS prevention that focused on educating clients on virology or safe sex did not attract as many Haitian clients, and those in attendance often remained silent. Irene's concerns about protecting her daughter and herself from unwanted disclosure, stigma, and harassment and about her immigration troubles, along with clients' willingness to respond with support and advice, indicate a desire for prevention programming that is holistic, encourages social relationships, and deals with immediate concerns.

As I showed in the previous chapter, HIV/AIDS prevention programs at many healthcare venues like Miami General and low- or no-fee health clinics were not well attended by Haitians for a variety of reasons, including affordability, convenience, poor treatment by providers, fear of being reported to authorities or being seen by other Haitians, and saturation with HIV-related issues. Health department training seminars for providers conducted in Kreyòl were not well attended either. The training manager for these seminars said that they consistently had to cancel the seminars because not enough people attended or were interested in attending seminars intended specifically for Haitians (that is, the seminars were in Kreyòl). These concerns indicate serious and complex misalignments between the ways in which experts, like Steve in the opening vignette, envision conducting HIV/AIDS prevention through the notion of community—as groups of people coming together on the basis of their shared disease and common risk—and how clients like Nadege, Magda, and Irene negotiate individual and collective participation and assembling in the name of science and public health.

The Politics of Community

By definition, the focus of public health is to "improve the health of communities" (Novick et al. 2008, 1). Public health has been viewed in contrast to biomedicine because it acts on population-level health issues and environmental determinants of health rather than on individual-level health issues. However, the biomedical model still dominates public health practice (Starr 2009). For instance, the social epidemiologist Nancy Krieger argues that public health, like biomedicine, "emphasizes biological determinants of disease amenable to intervention through the health care system, considers social determinants of disease to be at best secondary (if not irrelevant), and views populations simply as the sum of individuals and population patterns of disease as simply reflective of individual cases" (1994, 892). Public health prevention, as a result, has largely been a response to determinants of individual cases than to the determinants of population incidence rates. In other words, prevention is understood primarily through strategies focused on high-risk models, based on an individual's level of susceptibility, rather than through strategies to shift the distribution of disease throughout the population by actions such as mass environmental control or changing social norms (Rose 2007).

The biomedical model has remained generally accepted as the focus of public health practice continues to shift from curbing infectious disease epidemics and environmental threats to concentrating on the prevention of chronic diseases (such as cancer, heart disease, and stroke) and the maintenance of optimal health (through healthy diet and exercise, for example). Behavioral models emphasizing individual responsibility and choice remain essential components of prevention programs; programs focused on eliminating physical or infectious agents of disease through governmental regulation such as partner notification, quarantine, and disease reporting are important but secondary prevention strategies (Gostin et al., 1999).

HIV/AIDS represents a unique dilemma for public health prevention and highlights its inherent paradox. HIV/AIDS is both an infectious disease and a chronic condition. HIV/AIDS prevention consists of governmental oversight and control at the level of populations and communities as well as individually based behavioral and treatment interventions. Strategies for advancing HIV/AIDS prevention and expertise have revolved around treatment advances, testing initiatives, epidemiological and behavioral surveillance, increased access and linkage to care and treatment, case management, and risk reduction services. Much of HIV/AIDS prevention has focused on innovations aimed at decreasing an individual's risk for disease—as opposed to population-level changes—through clinically driven care and treatment, surveillance, and personal behavioral changes.

Over the years, as a result of research findings about the limitations of biological and behavioral interventions that concentrate solely on education, motivational changes, or treatment, public health advocates have called for an increased focus on broader sociocultural, political, and structural forces that contribute to group-level risk (Commission on Social Determinants of Health 2008; Herdt et al. 1991; Link and Phelan 1995; Marmot and Wilkinson 1999; Smedley et al. 2002). Leading health institutions have linked poor health outcomes to social and physical environmental factors as well as access to health services. They have also argued that some populations carry disproportionately heavier disease burdens than others, due to lack of opportunities and resources to maintain and improve health (Commission on Social Determinants of Health 2008; Frieden 2010; Marmot and Wilkinson 1999; Satcher 2006). And advancing the health of entire communities, or a population-based health perspective, has been a core component of the response to these calls for change. The paradox is that although public health prevention in this model emphasizes social, economic, and environmental interventions at the level of the community, experts in the field of HIV/AIDS prevention continue to act on communities through traditional high-risk strategies designed for individuals.

As I showed in chapter 2, HIV/AIDS prevention uses techniques of case-based surveillance and epidemiology to identify individual risk and then groups individuals together on the basis of this risk. For instance, groups center around behavioral characteristics associated with high risk such as men who have sex with men, intravenous drug users, and, more recently, heterosexuals. Other groups, like Haitians, are socially defined based on race and ethnicity, gender, age, education, and nationality. The characteristics that define these groups are conceptualized as distinct categories, and the groups themselves are conceptually flattened to seem as if they were naturally occurring categories of difference, even though they have varying logics, histories, and meanings. These groups, nevertheless, are the primary conduits through which we come to know, understand, and talk about HIV/AIDS prevention. They also have become the "communities" targeted by HIV/AIDS prevention and intervention programs and messages.

In popular, programmatic, and scholarly usage, these behaviorally and socially constructed categories that reflect individual calculations of risk have easily come to stand in for culturally distinct communities, with a shared history, social ties, practices, values, and beliefs that put them collectively at risk. The sociologist Steven Epstein calls this move "categorical alignment," in which politically or socially defined differences are mapped directly onto the differences that are the products of biomedical research (2010, 69). Culture can be effortlessly mapped onto these categories "as a set of natural character traits" that are ahistorical and atemporal (Jenks 2010, 212), because they are products of an individual-based approach to etiology and describe personal characteristics of individuals (such as their beliefs and attributes). As documented in the previous sections on the training workshops, HIV/AIDS prevention experts are inculcated to mediate and act on risk at the level of behavior (through promoting safe sex and routine testing, for example) and culture (such as using *oungans* to teach about condom use and seeing medical care as preventive). Culture becomes not only a way to decontextualize the complex formulations of how people see themselves in relation to others, but also a way to justify the lack of HIV/AIDS intervention and prevention programs for certain groups—for example, because Haitians are difficult to reach and reluctant to discuss HIV/AIDS. This has the effect of naturalizing risk as behaviorally, biologically, and culturally mediated.

Haitians' notions of community and culture are also complex and contested, and they differ from those of HIV/AIDS experts. Many Haitians told me that a Haitian community did exist, but they were unsure of whom or what this community consisted. Haitians spoke about how Haitian communities in Miami reflected those in Haiti. For instance, Claudette, the convenience store owner in Little Haiti, told me matter-of-factly: "Some [people are] close [to me], some not too close. That depends on when and where they come from in Haiti." Lara Pierre, a Haitian community activist who worked for a well-known Haitian social services agency in Miami, explained how practices that bind individuals together from the sense of shared familial or regional ties can also force individuals to make difficult choices in social conduct that may not be sanctioned by norms in the United States: "The most significant is where they came from in Haiti, because it really informs in a lot of other things that they do here, either self-perception, who they choose to trust, who they associate with, and how vulnerable they become because of this sense of solidarity with the group from the same area in Haiti. So say you need a car and you go to a particular person because you're kinfolk and he's from your home town, and it turns out that he ripped you off. And you don't want to go to the authorities because your mother and his mother go back a long way."

In a similar vein, other people described the community as being bound together by a common past of living in and leaving Haiti and by an uncertain future of facing similar problems of racial discrimination and marginalization in Miami. For instance, those living in the neighborhoods around Little Haiti said that daily social interactions, described as walking and talking with friends and neighbors freely and sitting out on the porch and listening to music, formed the mainstay of the notion of community because these daily activities were most reminiscent of life in Haiti. Many also described Little Haiti as a place for impoverished Haitians or as temporary residence for recent Haitian immigrants or refugees who would move to the suburbs of Miramar and Kendall as soon as they could afford to do so. Many Haitians felt that although these residential patterns based on economic divisions in Miami fractured the concept of community, they mirrored the way communities were stratified in Haiti.

Others talked about community in terms of a common future in Miami that was bleak for all Haitians. Christine Beaudet, a young woman who had just earned a degree at a two-year community college, told me: "It's like I don't like Miami; I really don't like it. It's really hard here for Haitians. The government . . . you know . . . Haitians have a lot of discrimination. I've learned that when I was in Haiti it was better but right now, it's really hard. I don't plan to stay in Miami because we don't get paid." Christine's friend, Brigitte Jeune, added: "I'm not too sure about being here either. Like the other day, me and my mom went to a hotel to look for a job for her and then the lady told her something like . . . 'Don't you know how lucky that you got a job?' It was like a housekeeping job. What is so lucky about getting a housekeeping job? I was like 'Lucky for what? Because she can't speak any English?'"

The notion of community among Haitians in Miami is not only rooted in conflict and contestation, but also born of it. These negative connotations associated with community become expressed as exclusive to the Haitian people due to a collective history of conflict and struggle. To many Haitians, a sense of an imagined community or nationalism (B. Anderson 1983; Creed 2004) failed to exist in Haiti and has never been resurrected in Miami. The anthropologist Michel-Rolph Trouillot (1990, 1995) attributes this failure in Haiti to the Haitian Revolution, in which Haitians led the only successful slave revolution in modern history—an event that historically has been largely ignored. He argues that the revolution created an independent modern state but not a nation. As a result, a shared collective developed more because of the existence of a common language, religious practices, and cultural models than because there were sustained projects of nation building and citizenship (Gros 2000; Trouillot 1990). These factors, along with long periods of internal political strife, foreign occupation, and forced economic and political isolation, have led to deep and complex societal divisions in Haiti (Gros 2000; Kumar 1998; Trouillot 1990).

Many Haitians in Miami expressed these divisions in rather mundane terms, saying that Haitians could not live together as a community—setting them apart from other ethnic communities in Miami, particularly Cubans. Richard Jaubert, an older man who frequented the HIV/AIDS classes at Miami General, explained that these kinds of divisions were rooted in systematic divisions in Haiti and continued to impede Haitians' economic and political success in Miami:

> The people who really look at Haitians the wrong way is the same Haitians, the same people. Haitian on Haitian. I don't believe the other nationalities are the same. The Cubans, if one person had a house, they always give a helping hand. That means if they have one place, one can just sleep here now and in a couple of hours, the other one come and get the bed and sleep so they help each other. They really live together; Haitians are not like that. They don't want to understand how to find a way to live together. That's the same system in Haiti. If a person has a dollar in his hand, he'll never give it to you. He sees nothing. My way is giving; I'm a giver, but Haitians—when you give them, it's like you owe them.

Here Richard, like many others, positions himself as other—someone who is a "giver," who is not like "them," not like other Haitians. He revokes his own group affiliation when he denies behaving in a way that is seen as representative of the Haitian community.

Many others felt that the potency of race and racism in the United States not only reinforced and exacerbated the social and economic divisions found in Haiti, but also structured the polarization between Cubans and Haitians. Junie Auguste, a Haitian HIV/AIDS counselor, reasoned that being seen (in both popular and official rhetoric) as "boat people," as uneducated and carriers of disease, made everyday acts of discrimination against Haitians normal. "Haitians have the stigma that we are boat people, that we are people mostly coming from boats, and that we don't know how to read, how to write, that we don't know anything about hygiene," she declared. "So we have a lot of stigma as the Haitian community that we have to try to get rid of, but it's difficult, and living in Miami is even worse because you have the Hispanic community which is well established here and the laws favor them. So we have to work probably four times as hard as the Hispanic community. It's well known and documented that when they do come by boats the way we do and they come from political and economic hardship the way we do, the laws favor them. The worse thing is that [discrimination] is not only blatant but normal. It's just normal, that's the thing." Junie asserts that the associations related to boat people are driven by immigration policies rooted in racial and ethnic prejudice, which reinforce Haitians' resentment of their own identity and bolster envy between Hispanics and Haitians in Miami. According to Junie, depictions of boat people as unhygienic and illiterate, and the racial discrimination and prejudice that undergird these depictions, have become naturalized pieces of the "Haitian" identity.

Mona Blanc, the Haitian patient advocate at Miami General, asserted that the tensions between Cubans and Haitians were embedded within existing racial and ethnic conflicts in the United States:

> When you look at it, it's not really the Cuban and the Haitian and the Haitian and the Cuban. It's what? It's like a mother or a father who have different children but those parents have one or two favorite children so what happens? Jealousy. Like if you go to the Bible, and remember Joseph was the favorite of his father. So what happened? They sell Joseph because they were jealous of Joseph. That is not really because Joseph was the fault; it's because their father favored Joseph over them. He was the little one, so I can understand spoiling the little one—so that's what happened. It's not really the Cuban and the Haitian. No! The Haitians are frustrated when they see that the Cuban come here, if the Cuban step on the ground, on the soil, they can stay. So when they see that . . . the Cuban come, I see that they swing over and they step by the beach and they stay. But the Haitian, they were sitting there by the bridge; they all were sitting there by the bridge. That means that they were not even on the beach; they come on land and sit by the bridge. They send them back anyway.

Mona recounts the story of Joseph in the Book of Genesis, how this favorite son of Jacob was sold into slavery by his jealous brothers. She reasons that it was the favoritism exhibited by Jacob that caused the rift between Joseph and his brothers, in much the same way that differential immigration policies, rooted in racism, create and sustain divisions between Haitians and Cubans in Miami.

Similarly, Henry Deveroux, a Haitian nonprofit administrator, explained the positioning of Haitians in Miami as part of a larger discourse surrounding the racialized landscape in Miami. He said: "Cubans control the majority of the political and economic power in Miami, and this breeds a lot of resentment for everyone else. They can also be more racist than whites, too. I personally think that the situation in Cuba and Haiti is the same: the political instability, the threat of death. But the United States considers them different, and that is based on prejudice. It's not as bad as it used to be, but it is still there. There is a lot of infighting, like between Jamaicans, African Americans, and Haitians, because there is very little power to grab onto for these groups, so they fight among themselves." Henry contends that due to racism and political and economic bias, Haitians are not granted certain political and economic resources allotted to other immigrant groups. He also declares that such racialized predicaments are a result of problems between different racial and ethnic minority groups, because so much time is spent fighting for limited resources.

Henry was not alone in his sentiments. Many informants told me that "Haitians can't see the bigger picture," meaning that Haitians' lack of effective leadership and civic engagement prevented them from developing broad social movements to improve economic and political equality. Jerome, the counselor at Sante Ayisyen, told me: "We are not a nation where we like to help each other, which is sad. Even though the laws favor people coming from Cuba, you have to admire them because they do stick together. They help each other. They are powerful politically because they elect each other. They make sure that they are part of the mainstream America politically, which is what we don't do. It's only recently that we are starting to do that, and even then you find people from the outside, like a Hispanic or a Caucasian, who come in and try to pit Haitians against each other." Jerome said that the lack of social ties that bind people together in Haiti extend to conditions in Miami; he also maintained that individual Haitians tend to ignore the group's political goals for personal gain.

Lara Pierre, the community activist, declared that these types of behaviors in Miami were due to "political baggage" from Haiti, where "dirty politics" were the root cause of a failed political system. She said that Haitians "don't understand that having enough Haitian elected officials will give power to everyone, and so it lowers the sum total of respect that people have for Haitians period because [people will start to think that] these people you know, they're not like the Hispanics . . . they hate each other, they hate themselves." The political scientist Jean-Germain Gros describes these political conflicts in Haiti as having a "kamikaze quality," where "short-term victories for a few and by any means necessary are pursued with zeal matched only by the certainty of defeat for Haiti as a country" (2000, 225). Lara's response, like those of Jerome, Richard, and Henry, indicates that lack of cohesiveness among Haitians both in Haiti and in Miami is entrenched in and sustained by damaged subjectivities, self-deprecation, and collective devaluation, all of which stems from a long history of dehumanizing racism and debilitating sociocultural and political marginalization (Fanon 1967; Gilman 1985, 1986).

When I asked about community cohesiveness and activism, many informants said that they were not involved in the Haitian community because of fear of deportation, possible violence to family members in Haiti, and perceptions that the community would not offer anything in return. Many Haitian clients were so fearful of being associated with projects related to Haitians that a few refused to be interviewed by me, often saying that they weren't "political." Even repeated pleas and explanations of my research seldom convinced them to participate. Lara, the community activist, said that it was "natural" for

Haitians to think that speaking to me was "political." She explained that this situation was part of a broader dilemma for those working in social activism as well: "We're always saying if you want to change the condition of your life, you really need to speak up, you really need to raise your voices to be heard . . . not in protest . . . just, you know, an expression, a vision of an idea of 'this is what I want for my community.' To them all of that is political, and all of that brings repercussions [of a negative kind]." Lara observed that the act of speaking or "being heard" in any way is political for many Haitians because it is rooted in the long and complex history of Haiti, where voicing personal sentiments often provoked severe retributions.

Self-described community activists like Lara feel that the political and economic position of Haitians in Miami had improved and was continuing to get better. She is part of a growing legion of Haitian activists promoting civic engagement among Haitian residents of Miami. She organized protests, demonstrations, and voting drives, initiatives that were part of a larger push for self-advocacy and self-reliance in the realm of health, politics, and labor. These undertakings strongly parallel public health campaigns, such as those related to HIV/AIDS prevention and intervention, that strive to make the individual responsible for his or her own health and well-being, often obscuring broader historical and social frameworks. Social activists like Lara have much in common with people who are not as optimistic about the future, those who continually point to the limited political and economic gains that Haitians in Miami have been able to realize, and even those who emphasize that Haitians are a "naturally" unpolitical and contentious community, an idea that is similar to their naturalization as diseased, poor, and suffering. Both the activists and those who are more pessimistic position Haitians as invariably caught between a "natural" proclivity for nonparticipation and their "cultural" baggage of strife and self-contempt.

Community, for both activists and Haitians in general, is experienced through intricate managements of extrication, indifference, and fidelity. It involves a double bind of allegiance, belonging conditionally to a community in Miami to which many don't wish to belong and remaining loyal to a community in Haiti that no longer exists, except for its legacy of misery, poverty, and injustice. Finally, community is lived simultaneously as vulnerability and resiliency—implying not necessarily powerlessness but surely unequal power.

From Experience to Expertise

HIV/AIDS prevention experts are continually encouraging their Haitian clients, both HIV-positive and HIV-negative, to be the "drivers" of their medical care, to "be empowered," and to see new "opportunities" in being HIV-positive. But these modern visions of patients are always already muted by constructions of a particular Haitian identity and collectivity as steeped in too much culture, too much ignorance, and too much hopelessness. Experts suggest that Haitians can shed and transcend such undesirable characteristics through the very principles of responsible citizenship—education, self-governance, and civic agency—that are routinely made inaccessible to them by everyday forms of racism and marginalization. Clients are fully implicated here as well. They continually orient themselves to various institutions or diseases, negotiate resources, and vie to live both inside and outside the system, while at the same time the system is generating data about the dangers of their particular group.

In documenting the relationship between the gay rights movement and HIV/AIDS activism, Epstein writes: "In the field of biomedicine, for example, certainly the patient who 'does her homework' and confronts her doctor with alternative perspectives about her own conditions is making a foray of sorts into the domain of lay participation. But when whole groups of patients suffering from the same disease establish new organizations, elaborate a collective sense of self, and then act in concert to challenge the medical conceptualizations of their condition and its treatment, then the intervention is potentially both more radical in character and more transformative in its consequences" (2003, 173). The story here is not an analysis of marginalized individuals' attempts at altering science from "below." Rather, it is an account of the multiple ways to conceptualize transformative social movements in health, especially in the absence of collective participation due to complex economic, political, and social disenfranchisement and history. Even in the so-called margins, there are several key sites of struggle and social participation, as Haitians in Miami engage in wider debates over expertise and community as both responsible citizens and unmanageable subjects.

4

Treating Citizens

The Promise of Positive Living

I met Jacques Chantal through his social worker, Miriam Spencer, at Miami General Hospital. Miriam characterized Jacques as a "successful" patient and an "ideal" person to answer questions about HIV/AIDS in the Haitian community. When we first met, Jacques—openly and without hesitation—told me that he was gay, in his late twenties, and in the country illegally, and that he had been HIV-positive for several years. He explained that he had come to the United States with his family legally as a young child but had then been deported to Haiti as a teenager for attempting to sell $20 of marijuana to an undercover policeman. He had known his HIV-positive status before he was deported. When his health began to deteriorate in Haiti, he returned to the United States illegally thanks to a technical error on the government's part, in order to have access to better medications and health care.

One hot morning in mid-July, I set out to accompany Jacques on a series of appointments with various social and medical institutions. The first appointment was to find out about affordable housing at Safe Haven, an organization that provided social and psychological services to the poor. Jacques was excited and eager to find out more about the independent housing options that they offered because he hated where he was currently staying: a residential facility for the homeless, where he had to endure frequent thefts of his belongings and aggressive harassment from other residents. He read the brochure about Safe Haven to me several times while I drove, as if he were trying to memorize the lines:

> Safe Haven offers a continuum of residential settings ranging from highly supervised group homes to more independent satellite apartments. All residences are integrated into the community. The members are assisted with skills associated with daily living, i.e. education regarding self-care living skills, interpersonal communication, personal hygiene, grooming

and tenant living skills. Staff give the residents the support and assistance necessary to help individuals become increasingly independent in community living. The goal is to provide safe, secure, and affordable housing to the individuals served. All residents must be employed or participate fully in the program, and must attend mandatory weekly guidance counseling.

Jacques told me repeatedly that his counselor thought that he would be "perfect" for this program because he was independent, employed, and a good patient.

When we arrived, we met with Sarah Hines, the program manager. She explained: "There is currently a waiting list for residence at Safe Haven. Jacques, you have to fill out an application and complete a health evaluation before being placed on the list." Jacques interrupted by asking, "Do you have any space in your homeless facility?" highlighting the insecurity of his current living situation. Very patiently, Sarah explained: "Our homeless facility is for homeless clients or for people in emergency situations." She repeated: "You have to fill out the application to get on the waiting list."

Sarah then asked questions about Jacques's past mental health disorder treatments, hospitalizations, and medications. When Jacques had responded "no" to each question, Sarah put her pen down, looked directly at him, and said: "This is strange, because most of the people that your counselor refers to me qualify, but if you don't have a history of psychiatric disabilities or disorders or are not diagnosed with anything, then we would have a problem with your qualifying." She added: "You may also want to think about whether this is something that you want to do. I mean, would you want to live in this kind of a facility? Some of our cases are pretty severe even in independent housing. I don't know if you would want to live there if you even qualified under mild depression." At this point, Jacques seemed completely dejected, nodding his head slowly. Then he quietly asked: "Is it still possible to fill out the application? Because I don't mind living there." Sarah politely repeated: "Please talk with your counselor and complete the psychosocial evaluation. I also want you think hard about living in a facility for those with psychiatric issues." We thanked her and left.

On the way to the car, Jacques broke our silence by complaining about his hunger. I offered him some extra food vouchers given out by pharmaceutical companies as incentives for attending clinical support groups for people infected and affected by HIV/AIDS. Because many Haitians who enrolled in HIV/AIDS intervention programs, like Jacques, had severe food insecurities, I usually saved the vouchers that I was given to distribute so they could purchase extra meals to take home. Jacques didn't discuss our visit while we were eating. As we got back in the car, however, I asked him about his thoughts on Sarah's description of life at Safe Haven. To me, her description seemed to mirror the brochure's depiction of a place designed to cultivate independence rather than to house people, like Jacques, who were seen as already independent. Because of Jacques's continuing silence, I sensed that the reality of his residential choices was sinking in. He had to decide between continuing to live in the homeless facility, where he faced the daily threat of robbery and harassment, and "proving" he had a psychiatric pathology to get on the waiting list for Safe Haven, essentially a facility for the mentally ill. Jacques stared out the window and said in a defeated voice: "I would still live there, but her questions made me wonder if it was really independent living."

After lunch, we headed off to visit his aunt, whom he described as a *mambo* (voodoo priestess) and the owner of a Haitian botanica. When we arrived, Jacques opened his notebook, took out a few twenty-dollar bills from his wallet, and told his aunt how to distribute it. She was leaving for Haiti the next day, and he wanted to send some of the money that he had made working as a server at restaurants to various family members and friends back in Haiti. He exclaimed: "Man, I have no more money because all of it went to Haiti!" He also gave her about twenty dollars to put toward his savings, money that was under her name since he could not legally open a bank account in the United States. He explained: "I don't do nothing, don't go out, buy anything. . . . I just do my thing, go to work, eat, sleep, so all my money goes to saving up . . . I guess for a lawyer."

Even though at the time people with HIV/AIDS were barred from entering the United States, Jacques had been diligently saving all of his money in the hope of getting an immigration attorney who could lobby for medical amnesty based on his HIV-positive status. He knew that he had received his current visa as the result of a government error, and he lived in constant fear that this error would be detected and he would be detained, deported, and deprived of medical care for his condition.

When we arrived at his last appointment of the day at Miami General Hospital, the attending physician read Jacques's name on the chart, looked him up and down, and said in surprise: "Are you Haitian? You speak perfect English." She went on to ask about his health and his CD4 counts. Jacques responded: "I'm feeling good. I've been taking all of my meds on time." He added: "Oh, but I did stop using that anal wart cream because Dr. Murray told me I could stop because I was getting a bad rash." The physician chided him like a child: "You know you are only supposed to stop using it for a couple of days and then go back to using it." She continued: "Have you seen a gastroenterologist?" Jacques looked confused and asked: "What is that?" When she explained, Jacques said, "Oh, yeah. They gave me a referral, but I couldn't schedule the appointment because the clinic nurses never called me back."

When the physician was finished, we went to the HIV/AIDS clinic so that Jacques could inquire about his referral. When staff members there asked him about names of physicians and reasons for the referral, Jacques indicated that he did not know: "Oh, I forgot her name. . . . She gave me a referral for—what's that thing where they put that thing and look inside you?" It was clear that this was not the first time they had heard something like this, since they managed to deduce within minutes that he needed a colonoscopy and wrote down the information for the referral.

Back in the car, he made a phone call for the referral. The person must have asked for his hospital card number, because he rifled through his wallet, exclaiming: "Oh shit! They didn't give me back the card." He explained that he couldn't get any medical or social services without this card and ran back to the hospital to find it. To both of our relief, he was able to locate the card. On the drive back, he reiterated how "terrified" he was about his legal uncertainties and that he was reluctant to hand over his savings to an attorney who would probably do nothing. He thanked me for driving, stating: "I would have never gotten all this stuff done without a car."

Jacques's situation is typical. Many Haitians, regardless of their HIV/AIDS status, must conduct complex negotiations in their daily encounters with various medical and social service institutions while trying to secure economic and health benefits in Miami. They experience barriers such as illiteracy, difficulty with the English language, and acute legal and economic uncertainties. Undocumented status, destitution, and severe personal isolation due to policies and practices that continue to marginalize Haitians force many of them into difficult and often hazardous situations related to their health and living conditions. Even Jacques, hailed by his providers as an "ideal," "successful" and "model" HIV/AIDS patient due to his self-reliance and medical compliance, faces significant struggles due to his tenuous immigration status and housing and food insecurity, as well as local and public health perceptions of Haitians as uneducated disease carriers and the various institutional assessments of vulnerability that accompany citizenship and social welfare projects.

In this chapter, I first focus on how individuals like Jacques come to embody the notion of "positive living," a key component of HIV/AIDS prevention programming that emphasizes self-sufficiency, medical compliance, and personal empowerment vis-à-vis HIV/AIDS. Second, I outline how positive living operates in HIV/AIDS programs in Miami. Specifically, I address (1) how positive living is linked to broader illness-based identity movements that emphasize empowerment, self-improvement, and self-transformation in the face of living with disease; (2) how it is a concept in which responsibility for one's self coexists and overlaps with responsibility to various others; (3) how it delineates and is characterized by a set of practices that form the foundation of HIV/AIDS prevention (adherence, disclosure, and safe sex); and (4) how its concept and strategies are fundamentally those of what scholars call "biological citizenship," a set of new dynamic relations among biology, rights-based politics, and identity. Bringing the discourses of biological citizenship into the context of how positive living functions in HIV/AIDS programs helps us see the ways in which it is neither a direct reapplication of nationally located ideas of social citizenship nor a radical departure from them.

For Jacques and many other Haitians in Miami, positive living is not always possible due to continuing legacies of punitive immigration, economic, and social policies that reinforce Haitians' position as natural disease carriers, illegal economic refugees, and unequal citizens. Even in describing some Haitians as model patients and citizens who represent the ideal of positive living, providers and programs downplay Haitians' daily struggle to survive. Jacques's providers, for instance, often highlighted his stellar medical compliance and unwavering commitment to institutional interventions, while failing to acknowledge his desperate struggles to evade arrest and deportation and to overcome discrimination, hunger, poverty, and homelessness. Jacques, in turn, negotiates critical resources and strategically navigates through myriad political, social, and medical bureaucracies by simultaneously claiming and rejecting biological citizenship and positive living projects. In their daily struggles, Haitians in Miami articulate the potency of exclusionary national politics within public health interventions and within the realm of biological citizenship.

Narratives of Empowerment and Transformation

"Positive living" is a movement that has become synonymous with HIV/AIDS in recent years. As those with HIV/AIDS live longer through the use of antiretrovirals and better managed care, activists and providers seek to change the focus of being HIV-positive from dying to living with disease, and they do this through the rhetoric of empowerment. As one community-based organization in Florida put it, "the challenge is no longer HIV itself; instead, the challenge is how to take control of one's own life, acknowledge the difficulties, face each day with renewed hope, and live with the reality that no one is alone in this battle" (Okaloosa AIDS Support and Informational Services 2007).[1] Many positive living programs in the United States, like the North Carolina Council for Positive Living, focus on issues of personal, social, and medical empowerment through programs that endorse activism and health literacy. Others designed for global settings, like the US Agency for International Development's Positive Living Project in Nigeria, emphasize economic development, extended health care, capacity building, and prevention.

Increasingly central to positive living in HIV/AIDS are concepts of empowerment, self-improvement, consciousness-raising, and advocacy for social change, all of which are inherently grounded in a biomedical framework. The mission of positive living stems from a confluence of events: previous self-help and rights-based movements, the increasing medicalization of daily life, and the growing focus on health promotion (Andrews 1993; Coreil and Mayard 2006; Lyttleton 2000; MacLachlan 1992; H. Matthews 2000; Robins 2006). For instance, HIV/AIDS-based movements, much like other illness-based identity movements, represent people's responses to the unpredictable nature of risk and their distrust of biomedical expertise (Coreil and Mayard 2006; Robins 2006). Early HIV/AIDS activists in the United States, concerned by governmental indifference and the exclusionary practices of biomedical research, sought to gain entry as credible participants in the production and dissemination of HIV/AIDS knowledge (Epstein 1996). Their success was partly a result of their ability to mobilize effective educational programs, self-help groups, and counseling and treatment strategies long before governmental public health involvement (Epstein 1996; MacLachlan 1992). The HIV/AIDS activist John MacLachlan writes that "the trend has been towards structures and control mechanisms based on the urge to deal with AIDS as a social problem, as a problem of consolidation of the AIDS organizations and their professional elite, and a problem of resource allocation, management, and control by the policy-makers" (1992, 454). These early initiatives, spearheaded largely by gay white men, were founded on the principles of gay consciousness-raising and centered on the importance of empowerment, autonomy, control over one's own life, the exhumation of neglected gay history, and revealing the existence of prejudice and discrimination. Over time, however, the movement based on the self-help ethos transformed itself to include a variety of constituents affected by the disease, including racial and ethnic minorities and women.

Essential features of HIV/AIDS support groups such as counseling, education, and outreach include principles related to individual responsibility, self-help, and social justice that are entrenched in institutional ideals of treatment efficacy and scientific models of prevention. In an HIV/AIDS prevention education class conducted in Kreyòl at Miami General Hospital, for example, Jill Leverett (or Miss Jill, as we all called her), requested advice from fellow group members about a situation that had been troubling her. Miss Jill was a middle-aged woman and a single mother of a young son. I had recently helped her move from a dilapidated apartment complex in Little Haiti to a newly refurbished three-bedroom cottage on the outskirts of North Miami. Although she relied on public assistance, including food stamps, to help her make ends meet, she had saved diligently for years to be able to rent a single-family home. Moving to her own home, she told me, holding back tears, "is something that I thank God for every day."

In the class, Miss Jill told us that a few weeks before, she had received a letter displaying the words "HIV/AIDS" on the envelope. She felt "horrible" receiving such a letter at her home because the people she lived with did not know that she was HIV-positive. She didn't feel that it was "right" for anyone to send such a letter to her home with "those words written on the outside for everyone to see." Mona Blanc, a Haitian hospital volunteer and newly minted patient educator, peered at Miss Jill and the rest of us from over the top rims of her thick glasses. She told Miss Jill in an unsympathetic and stern voice to "take responsibility" and to "call where the letter comes from." Mona reminded Miss Jill to demand to talk to someone who spoke Kreyòl and to insist on a translator if there wasn't one available.

Mona always addressed group members' questions and concerns with a Haitian proverb and related story. In response to Miss Jill's problems, Mona declared "chita pa bay," which she translated as "the more we stay in our corner, the less we learn." She explained: "You should not wait too long to ask someone for something that you need." She told us a story: "This lady went to her neighbor and started describing her money problems, taking all day to sit and talk. While this woman was visiting with her neighbor, she witnessed many people entering her neighbor's front door and asking for money. Her neighbor handed out cash to each and every one of these people that came. The end of the day approached, and the needy woman finally asked her neighbor for the ten dollars to feed her children. Her neighbor cried, surprised and annoyed, 'What? That's what you wanted all this time! Why didn't you just ask me earlier? See that woman who just came by? I just gave her $20 for the movies.'" Mona's audience replied with nodding, moans of understanding, and sighs of agreement. Mona insists on Haitians' right to demand medical privacy and language translation, stressing notions of self-responsibility and self-management. Her story is not so much about HIV/AIDS as it is about the proactive, assertive person who seeks out and obtains needed medical and social resources and challenges institutional roadblocks.

Immediately after Mona finished her story, Jaime Silva, the Hispanic lead health educator and a huge proponent of positive living, began to lecture on the importance of taking "the negativity of having a devastating disease and turn[ing] it into something positive." Jaime, who is HIV-positive and has an HIV-positive child, walked to the blackboard at the front of the class and wrote and underlined the words "positive" and "negative." He then wrote "love" under "positive" and "fear" under "negative." He said: "Humans have the power of choice and that they can choose which path to follow. We can either choose the positive path or the negative path, but when it often comes to disease, we choose the negative path of fear because of a lack of education and fear of discrimination and stigma."

Returning to his original dichotomy of "positive" and "negative" ways of thinking about disease, he asked the class members what the notion of "disease" meant to us. People responded by saying "deadly," "unhealthy," "virus," and "depression." Jaime nodded his head rapidly, as if these were the exact answers he wanted to hear. He explained that most people associate disease with "something negative," and that the key was to "turn this way of thinking into positive things." Mona interjected: "Yes, having a disease can give you a new beginning by giving you an opportunity to be healthy and to take care of yourself." Jaime continued: "Yes, like a crossroads, where you become more goal-oriented by taking control of your life and yourself by taking your medications, going to the doctor, and challenging yourself to keep on track. It can give people a lot of hope and can push people into being more responsible. You should present yourself at all times in a positive and powerful way."

Jaime and Mona both incorporate biomedical models of prevention into self-help approaches by teaching that testing positive for an incurable disease, in this case HIV/AIDS, is equivalent to personal and biological rebirth. Their approaches differ, however, in that Mona addresses the broader struggles that plague Haitians, regardless of their disease pathology. Mona's story teaches other Haitians how to overcome institutional hurdles such as a lack of medical privacy and access to language translation. In contrast, Jaime argues that an HIV-positive person should be thankful, gracious, and actively benevolent for being a beneficiary of such a transformative life experience. Like those of many providers and programs, his positive living narrative is one of blame, insinuating that it is only through an HIV-positive diagnosis that Haitians are able to take control of their lives and be "push[ed] . . . into being more responsible." Jaime fails to acknowledge the daily social and economic struggles that are critical to his clients, understanding them and their struggles only through the lens of their disease.

HIV/AIDS providers like Jaime also teach individuals that personal empowerment goes hand in hand with models of medical compliance. Many clients, in turn, regularly spoke of their life with HIV/AIDS using self-empowerment narratives that were rooted in scientific models of prevention, often minimizing the importance of the social context of HIV/AIDS. For instance, Tanesha Williams, an African American woman in a prevention education class conducted in English, declared:

> In order to live for a long time, you have to educate yourself, be strong, talk your mind, and take care of yourself because only you can do this, and nobody else, not even your doctor. It took me a long time to make inner peace with myself, and now I am thankful for the disease because I feel that I finally appreciate life and see it as a second chance. Don't just live but thrive! I take my medications, see my doctor, and come to these classes and support groups all the time. I live with this thing called HIV. HIV doesn't live with me. HIV doesn't control me. HIV is not my biggest

problem. You can't really just sit by and get down on the disease because you don't have time to do it. Look at me, I am normal, someone who stayed at home, did nothing but take care of my kids, went to church, did [Parent Teacher Association], and am God-fearing. My friends are angry that someone like me is a victim of the disease. I am a victim, but I am not angry and I don't let that stop me from going on with my life and living it the best I can.

Tanesha asserts her medical and moral adherence to the positive living movement by invoking her triumph over HIV/AIDS through the notions of choice, control, and compliance, declaring that it is she who "lives" with HIV/AIDS. Like Jaime and Mona, Tanesha attests to the promissory nature of positive living, realized through new ways of being and becoming empowered vis-à-vis HIV/AIDS. In her narrative, she indicates that there is an inherent injustice in her plight as a normal, church-going, God-fearing, and Parent Teacher Association mom who was infected with HIV/AIDS through no fault of her own. But this sentiment is overshadowed by her representation of positive living as both a biological and personal rebirth, an experience that transformed her from an angry victim into an appreciative strong woman living with HIV/AIDS. Individuals like Tanesha and Jacques are seen as models of positive living because they exhibit self-awareness and knowledge about the disease and its various attributes, and about everyday life in general. They also employ practices of transformation and humility predicated on performing medical compliance through the routine behaviors of treatment adherence and interaction with health care providers. Implicit in this conceptualization of so-called models of positive living is a downplaying of their concerns that are not related to disease, such as social stigma and housing insecurity.

Self and Social Responsibility

Individual responsibility within the framework of positive living goes hand in hand with social responsibility to various others, including sexual partners and those living with HIV/AIDS. First, many HIV/AIDS programs in Miami convey ideals of positive living as a means of exercising greater responsibility and honesty toward sexual partners. There is a strong sense that one has an uncontested responsibility not to spread the disease to others. For instance, a patient advocate in an educational class explained: "I would never want to infect anyone else because I would never want the things that happened to me to happen to anyone else. Remember that day that you found out? I wouldn't want anyone else to have that feeling ever in their lives, even though now I feel blessed with all the things that are going on in my life." This advocate expresses her unwillingness to have anyone else go through the experience of being HIV/AIDS positive, even though she herself feels "blessed" as a result of her disease. The concept of positive living implies a transformative process for the self through disease, coupled with an inherent moral mandate to prevent its spread to intimate partners—especially those who are not HIV-positive.

This accountability to others does not end with sexual partners; it includes a broader responsibility to all those living with HIV/AIDS. Both pharmaceutical company representatives and providers often state that all clients in prevention and treatment safety-net programs were lucky to receive antiretrovirals and other medications for free or for a modest fee. For instance, a nurse lectured a client who complained of the rising cost of medications: "It's a beautiful thing that you can get meds for free. Many people in the world don't have meds, and they would do anything for this opportunity." Many providers, like this nurse, often reiterate the good fortune and luck of HIV-positive clients in obligatory terms, using both moral and scientific frameworks without acknowledging why these clients are in need of free medications in the first place. That is, they instruct clients to faithfully adhere to their antiretroviral medication regimens because of their life-saving and life-giving properties that are not afforded to others; but they do so without addressing the extreme poverty that qualifies these clients for free medication. Nonadherence to medication is strongly linked to a lack of responsibility for one's own self and health. It is also associated with a blatant disregard for others who provided the opportunity for such drugs (that is, pharmaceutical companies, patient advocates, and social and health services providers) and for other patients who are denied this benefit.

Providers also implicitly connect this kind of social responsibility to HIV/AIDS advocacy and activism more broadly, especially when working with African Americans and Haitians because these two groups are seen by providers in Miami to be the least involved in garnering resources and support for various HIV/AIDS issues. For example, during an HIV/AIDS education class, an African American man named Chris Roberts commented that "society has blinders on over their eyes, mufflers over their ears, and a gag over their mouth," referring to the public's reluctance to increase aid to people living with HIV/AIDS. He exclaimed: "Whenever you turn on the TV, all you see is all those people with the 'Stop Abortion' signs and they are protesting, and what if we could have millions of people going to Washington for us? Nobody cares about AIDS."

Chris's statements did not go over well with Ramon Medina, a Hispanic social worker. Ramon responded by asking Chris: "How long have you had the disease?" Chris replied: "I was diagnosed last year in May." Ramon jumped in before Chris finished: "And before then, what did you know about AIDS and what did you do about AIDS?" Calm in the face of Ramon's outburst, Chris replied: "I didn't know nothing about the disease until I got it." Without acknowledging Chris's statements about public complacency in the United

States about HIV/AIDS, a disease that disproportionately affects racial and ethnic minorities, or his relative ignorance about HIV/AIDS despite abundant prevention programs, Ramon shouted at Chris and the rest of the class members, a few of whom were Haitians and the rest of whom were African Americans. Ramon said:

> There were a lot of people who fought for what you have, Chris. There are a lot of people who died for you. Many people went to Washington and tied themselves to flagpoles so that we could have the medication that we have today. What I think is the problem is that activism is not taken seriously right here in this room. When everything is gone is when you'll start complaining. People like you are complacent and just don't care about being advocates for budget cuts and for more services for AIDS patients. So when you want to complain about how you don't have this or that or when this and that is getting cut, you have no one to blame but yourself!

A couple of women indicated their support for Ramon by murmuring, "Tell 'em, Ramon!," but the majority of the audience was left speechless by his outburst. The tension was somewhat relieved by a woman who talked of the difficulties of raising children who are HIV-positive and traveling to Washington, D.C., to advocate for children's issues. Following her lead, the patient educator who was responsible for leading the class quickly steered the conversation away from activism.

Ramon's tirade is similar to other providers' lectures about complacency and the general lack of activism among African Americans and Haitians that do not discuss why these groups may not be engaged in public activism related to their HIV-positive status. Providers and patient activists continually use the positive living framework in these interventions to link advocacy and activism to the moral obligations of being HIV-positive and their attempts to build biosocial communities, groupings solidified on the basis of people's biological affliction (Rabinow 1992). In other words, if one is HIV-positive, one should be involved with other HIV-positive people in making sure that services and support are available for future generations and that resources are maintained for those currently in need. Clients are told that in order to be "effective advocates," they must be extremely knowledgeable about HIV/AIDS, unwaveringly focus on getting results, and have a strong rapport with others. In order to start on the path toward advocacy, clients are encouraged to have respect for themselves, others, and the cause.

In his outburst, Ramon accuses both Chris and the rest of the class of complacency and indifference because they do not take activism "seriously." Ramon presupposes Chris's obligation to act as an active and responsible recipient of health and social benefits as a result of his biological affliction (with HIV/AIDS). Ramon sees Chris's failure to act as indicative of his passivity, negligence, and blame-worthiness for the potential loss of HIV/AIDS resources for all current and future HIV-positive individuals. Ramon depicts Chris's inaction as a moral failure to fully recognize the stakes of his biological affliction, of a life lived with HIV/AIDS and the sacrifices embedded in such an acknowledgement. By marking African Americans and Haitians as people who exhibit persistent moral failures to act, providers reinforce notions of pathological dependence and passivity that result from and lead to social difference (of race and class). Providers and programs link African Americans and Haitians to diseases by which they have been routinely stigmatized, marking them as dependent and in perpetual need of governance, as well as unethical and undeserving recipients of resources, by erasing the social and political concerns at stake for these communities.

Reconceptualizing Positive Living

These notions of positive living and of responsibility to self and others were often not taken up by Haitian clients, activists, and providers as they were intended to do. Among Haitians, "positive living" was reinterpreted as a way to increase motivation and strength for caring for one's self and the group, without a direct link to any biological affliction. For instance, at a luncheon to celebrate World AIDS Day, Pierre Dumas, a young Haitian American spoken-word artist, applauded the "positiveness of people, especially those with HIV, who have so much hope and praise and who provide inspiration for the rest of the world." Simone Claude, another young Haitian activist, encouraged "people to feel positive and to be strong, and being positive gives you license to live stronger than ever and to never give up." Although neither Pierre nor Simone revealed their HIV status in their speeches, they conveyed the idea that living positively was a model for all Haitians to follow, regardless of their HIV status. Haitian activists and providers, like Mona in the section above, often adopted positive living as a way to teach Haitians how to approach the daily struggles of life in Miami as a marginalized community. However, positive living was delinked from biological affliction and reenvisioned as a means by which Haitians—an economically, politically, and socially marginalized community—could renew their hope for better lives in the present and future.

Haitian clients, activists, and providers also used three core strategies of scientific models of prevention—disclosure, adherence, and safe sex—to reconceptualize the official discourses of positive living. First, disclosing one's HIV status to others is considered a significant HIV/AIDS prevention strategy because it is seen as something that will potentially lead to safer sex behaviors (Pinkerton and Galletly 2007), better overall health outcomes (Stirratt et al. 2006), and increased social support (Serovich et al. 2000). In my discussions with Haitian clients, I heard many stories of relatives and friends who had responded to the disclosure of their HIV-positive status with rejection, abandonment, and even violence. Going against what was commonly taught in HIV/AIDS prevention classes, Mona counseled other Haitians who were HIV-positive to "think about disclosing carefully," instructing them to conceptualize disclosure as a "choice" rather than something one has to do. She emphasized that disclosure was not an obligation, and that one should weigh the positive and negative consequences of disclosing ("*sa bon oubyen sa pa bon*") to anyone, even intimate partners. During an HIV/AIDS intervention program for African Americans in which the discussion focused mainly on disclosure as representing "taking control" and "not being ashamed" of one's disease, Mona was the only Haitian present, and she continually spoke against such reasoning. She recounted a personal situation as an example for the class:

> For me, disclosing can't be done in the same way to different people. This is because each person is different, and sometimes it's important to pay attention to certain people before you feel comfortable disclosing to them. I don't have a problem disclosing but I could not disclose to my daughter for a long time. Just the other day, I was at church where very few people know about my status. There is a man at my church who is positive but he hasn't told anyone. He was bringing over his girlfriend to my house, and when my church friend, who did not know about me [being positive] but knew about him, found out about this and said to me, "Oh, don't let them drink out of your cup," I knew then that I would not feel comfortable disclosing to this person.

Consistent with research that indicates that disclosure is a distinct and complicated process that is dependent on the situation, context, and relationship (Cusick and Rhodes 1999; Mayfield Arnold et al. 2008), Mona, like many other Haitians, sees disclosure as a complex series of strategic procedures. For her, each act of disclosure has to be thoroughly evaluated and is dependent on systematic assessments of people and situations. Mona disagrees with the idea that disclosure is a means of taking control or showing pride—a common view in HIV/AIDS prevention programs—by framing it as careless and foolhardy through a series of stories that serve to showcase the extensive deliberation needed in each case of disclosure.

The conceptualization of disclosure as a complicated procedure among Haitian clients is fundamental to understanding their lack of openness about their HIV status. Although Jacques was open with me about his status, it is rare to encounter an HIV-positive Haitian client who declares his or her status publicly, even among other HIV-positive Haitians. Even HIV-positive

Haitian providers who were adept at teaching HIV-positive clients about living without shame had difficulty participating publicly in HIV/AIDS issues. For instance, Thomas Raymond, a young Haitian American social worker who was HIV-positive, explained that he would never participate in community caucuses or local policy-making committees, even though he had been a lifelong activist for HIV/AIDS issues. When I told him that I had been regularly attending local HIV/AIDS policy committee meetings and thought it would be beneficial to have someone like him advocating for issues relevant to other HIV-positive Haitians, he conveyed his surprise. "I could never ever stand up and tell people that I hardly knew that I am HIV-positive," he exclaimed. "This isn't because I am not an activist or committed to the issues, because I've always been involved. It's just that the assumption is outrageous, that you have to declare your status to be part of the decision-making process." Just as Mona insisted on evaluating each disclosure situation carefully, Thomas contradicted Ramon's assumption that not fully acting as an advocate and acknowledging a biological affliction publicly is a failure to enact social change related to HIV/AIDS. For Thomas and Mona, strategies related to the disclosure of an HIV-positive diagnosis had broader implications for Haitians in Miami in the context of their historical legacy of being labeled as an HIV/AIDS risk group. Their vision of positive living, much like that of the Haitian activists at the World AIDS Day celebration, signified living with hope and pride without an association to biological affliction.

In addition to questions about disclosure, Haitian clients and providers also translated the discourses of treatment adherence differently. In HIV/AIDS prevention programs, adherence was symbolic of individual self-reliance, self-sufficiency, and, as a patient educator put it, "of know[ing] your disease and how to fight it." Haitian providers and advocates spoke of treatment adherence in terms of medical compliance and taking medications consistently; they also used narratives of self-acceptance, self-trust, and assertiveness to showcase how to navigate life as a Haitian. For example, Louise Paulin, a Haitian nurse who routinely lectured Haitian clients in prevention classes on the importance of adherence, declared:

> Adherence means patience: patience to understand and to let the medication take its time in effectively working for you; patience with yourself in trying out and accepting medication and the disease. Adherence also means communication with your provider. This is crucial to adherence. You have to be open and direct with them, not only in listening to directions and advice but also give back, trust yourself in knowing your body and report any inconsistencies back to the doctor. Adherence also means to write notes which mean that you have to keep records of your physical well-being and to also be alert to yourself. You have to be careful and to

pay attention and, most of all, trust yourself more. There should be someone at the pharmacy or doctor's office who should explain these things to
you in Kreyòl and if there is not, make sure to have someone or to go to
someone that could translate for you.

Louise presented adherence as being not about the physical act of ingesting
antiretrovirals regularly, but about patience, assertiveness, open and direct
communication, record keeping, self-trust, and self-awareness. Adherence has
come to represent not only the transformations of self that are needed to accept
medications, diseases, and one's life situation, but also a way of knowing and
communicating about the suffering body of individual Haitians and Haitians as
a collective.

Finally, safer sex after a HIV-positive diagnosis was an important standard
within the paradigm of positive living. Having safe sex—or, more accurately,
using condoms and other forms of protection—is a fundamental part of many
intervention and prevention programs. In classes and workshops in Miami,
people who were HIV-positive were often told that having safe sex is "normal"
and a "good thing," with many providers and educators encouraging and promoting sex after an HIV-positive diagnosis. For instance, during a class titled
"Sex for Positives," a health educator declared: "You have to [have sex] physi-
cally because the need is biological, because your body has to release the fluids;
otherwise it's bad for you."

Many Haitian providers, however, rarely endorsed these ideas about having sex. Much like their Haitian clients, Haitian providers repeatedly advocated
the values of abstinence, monogamy, and fidelity. Mona, the patient educator,
took pride in claiming that many Haitians practiced abstinence after receiving
a HIV-positive diagnosis. When I asked if this was true of those in the Kreyòl
education class, every person nodded to indicate "yes." Renée Mevs said: "I have
a husband, but everybody sleep in their own bed. I have no interest. As soon
as you get virus, you shouldn't have sex. . . . I feel like that." Helen Joseph commented that she had similar sentiments after finding out that she was HIV-
positive, explaining that "I get a disgusting feeling when I think about sex. My
husband gave it to me, and I feel bad with life when I found out for a long time.
But now I've given my life to God." Richard Jaubert said: "I know I'm sick. I don't
like to transmit to others." Janvier Savain told us that she didn't want to tell anyone that she was HIV-positive, and Justine Jean-Phillipe expressed similar sentiments: "I have been abstinent for three years, and I feel lonely and depressed.
But I don't want to give it to someone else. I believe that according to viral load,
I'm undetectable, but I believe that if I had sex, the virus might flare up."

For these individuals, the absence of sexual and physical intimacy was an
accepted and expected result of their HIV-positive status, both because of their
fears about worsening their physical condition and transmitting the disease to

others, and because sex itself was a painful reminder of how they had become infected. It also signaled a reaction to the long time that they and other Haitians had been perceived negatively as disease carriers because of their biology, with the avoidance of all sexual practices serving to negate this biological representation. HIV/AIDS is often touted by providers and programs as not a moral issue, and full disclosure of one's HIV-positive status to sexual partners has become the gold standard of ethics. By viewing HIV/AIDS as a purely biological affliction in HIV/AIDS programs, providers seek to erase the association between HIV/AIDS and the so-called immoral behaviors that lead to contracting the disease. But these same providers and programs reinscribe morality as the dominant framework through which behavioral interventions, particularly those centered on positive living, are implemented. For many Haitian clients, the denial of sexual and physical intimacy represented the bypassing of disclosure altogether. The choice of abstinence served to symbolically negate and reject the practices through which infection occurred in the first place, to protect the individual from the potential negative consequences of disclosure, and to decouple biological association and national identity.

Haitian clients, advocates, and providers reinterpreted self-help and social empowerment ideals within positive living as tools for better living for all Haitians. Using the discourses about a set of biosocial practices—including disclosure, adherence, and safe sex—they shifted the focus of positive living to include notions of transformation and positive thinking that were not rooted in biological and risk-based conceptions of disease or scientific models of prevention. Positive living became a means of focusing on nonbiological struggles. Against the backdrop of long-standing negative stereotypes as disease carriers and of political, economic, and social disenfranchisement, positive living was repositioned as a way for Haitians to manage various citizenship and social welfare projects' assessments of their vulnerability and secure economic and social benefits.

Rethinking Biological Citizenship and Biosociality

Notions of individual responsibility and self-management that define the positive living movement represent what many have increasingly called biological citizenship (Ginsburg and Rapp 1995; Nguyen 2005; Petryna 2002; Rose 2007; Rose and Novas 2005). Biological citizenship is seen as an emerging form of citizenship, one that goes beyond the traditional notions of citizenship based on civil, social, and political rights; it reflects the needs and demands of citizens for social, economic, and political inclusion, as well as the recognition of new social identities in the growing spheres of biopolitics, biotechnology, and biomedicine. The anthropologist Adriana Petryna, in her study of the Ukraine's quest after the Chernobyl disaster to establish state legitimacy and autonomy through the creation of social welfare organizations to mitigate the consequences of the disaster, describes biological citizenship as "a massive demand for but selective access to a form of social welfare based on medical, scientific and legal criteria that both acknowledge biological injury and compensate for it" (2002, 6).

Expanding on Petryna's work, the sociologists Nikolas Rose and Carlos Novas used the term "to encompass all those citizenship projects that have linked their conceptions of citizens to beliefs about the biological existence of human beings, as individuals, as families and lineages, as communities, as population and races, and as a species" (2005, 440). Rose and Novas (2005) and Rose (2007) argue that although biological considerations have long shaped many aspects of citizenship, a new form of biological citizenship is materializing in the wake of expanding biotechnological and genomic innovations. They write:

> As aspects of life once placed on the side of fate become subjects of delib-
> eration and decision, a new space of hope and fear is being established
> around genetic and somatic individuality. In the nations of the West—
> Europe, Australia, and the United States—this is not taking the form
> of fatalism and passivity, and nor are we seeing a revival of genetic or
> biological determinism. Whilst in the residual social states in the post-
> Soviet era, biological citizenship may focus on the demand for financial
> support from state authorities, in the West novel practices of biological
> choice are taking place within a "regime of the self" as a prudent yet
> enterprising individual, actively shaping his or her life course through
> acts of choice. (Rose and Novas 2005, 458)

Rose and Novas argue that contemporary biological citizenship represents new ways of thinking about subjectivities, ethics, and politics due to vast changes in the ways that we have come to know the human body. In the age of genomics, human bodies are increasingly seen as exploitable and consumable objects that are fragmented and can be retooled and reshaped by various biotechnologi-cal innovations; these bodies are beyond the realm of national politics. People become increasingly seen as biological consumers, and not as traditional citi-zens who are bound to nation-states by rights and duties. Contemporary biolog-ical citizenship is seen to move away from eugenics and biosocial categories of difference (for example, age, gender, and race) that have shaped ideas of social and political citizenship in Western Europe since the mid-twentieth century. Biological citizenship, therefore, is seen as a radical shift toward an increasing interest in promoting active biological consumerism and individual well-being within "a political economy of hope" (Rose and Novas 2005, 442).

Although these discourses of biological citizenship do help us understand the complex links between biology and subjectivity, the concept of biological citizenship does not adequately capture the array of citizenship practices in the West, especially concerning economically, socially, and politically marginalized groups. It overlooks the ways in which biomedical innovation, knowledge, and interventions affect prevailing notions of difference and social hierarchy. It also offers very little to help us understand how ideas about categories of difference, such as race and sexual orientation, fuel practices that selectively alter and regulate individuals and populations. The narratives on positive living offer the possibility of expanding the conversation on biosociality and biological citizenship. We live in a time where the enduring influence of the state (through public health interventions) exists simultaneously with self-governance and individual responsibility. Positive living examples also focus our attention on the severe inequalities that ground our relationship to biotechnological endeavors.[2]

In Miami a large majority of recipients of HIV/AIDS programming are Haitians and others who are severely disenfranchised and who use their biological affliction to demand institutional economic, political, and social resources that are otherwise unavailable or unobtainable. For instance, Irene Dorval, the young Haitian HIV-positive single mother with an HIV-positive daughter, explained her daily struggle to make ends meet for her daughter and herself in the context of a discussion regarding community problems. She announced: "I have something to say! Money is the problem. I got a $1,000 a month from the social worker but it's not enough at all for all the things I got to pay for, like my bills, housing, cleaning supplies, food, clothing for my daughter. My social worker told me that I got HIV not AIDS, so I can't get more benefits. I am very angry about it. Isn't it discrimination that people with AIDS get more than me and the [other] people with just HIV? Don't I suffer the same? Don't I take the same medication? Don't I struggle the same with the disease? We can't live on this!" Irene argues that she, as someone categorized as HIV-positive, has the right to the same amount of resources given to someone who has AIDS because their suffering is the same. For Irene, her disease confers tremendous potential value and becomes the basis of claims for economic compensation; her argument also depicts a broader illustration of suffering and exclusion that is not rooted in biology.

For many clients, these resources are not limited to governmental monetary or health benefits but also include various forms of social and political inclusion. For instance, Mona Blanc, the patient educator, was hailed by providers and patients as a model of positive living, like Jacques Chantal. Mona had come to Miami General close to death over a decade ago, finding out that she had full-blown AIDS, but after several years she was hired as a clinical patient advocate and educator. Although I first met Mona at the hospital where she worked, I spent more time with her at her townhouse in North Miami Beach, where she lived with her elderly mother and her teenage daughter.

Like many other Haitians in Miami, Mona had traveled there through many other locales, including the Virgin Islands, Puerto Rico, New York, and Boston. She had been living in Miami for twenty-five years and often talked about how many changes she had witnessed during this time. Some things had gotten easier, such as navigating low-cost healthcare; some had gotten harder, like accessing reliable transportation. Mona constantly spoke of being positive, saying: "I like to be around positive people, positive thoughts, positive energy because I know energy travels so I have a group of people that I like to be around because I am trying to be positive all my life. I'm trying to go higher, so I don't like living around people who drag me down." She also had very different concepts about how to engage with Haitian clients than her colleagues at Miami General. She explained:

> Let's say that if you want to come to preach the gospel to someone who is hungry, the first thing that you should do is give them food, and then tell them that Jesus is alive or there is a God. The person is very hungry and you come and tell them about Jesus, and they are gonna tell you to get outta here and tell you they hungry. The sex thing is not the number one thing; the shooting drug is not the number one. They need other stuff. If we can give them something, like I was talking about, work permit, allow them to go to work, then you will talk to them about prevention, they will hear you because they say, "Oh, we care about this."

In addition, she made sure to remind everyone that the main reason Haitians didn't engage with prevention programs and Haitian-oriented health clinics was because of the perceived lack of confidentiality practiced by Haitian providers:

> Do you know how a lot of Haitians are dying just because they don't want to face another Haitian nurse or Haitian doctors? I had a friend of mine. She used to go to Miami General, and she had a problem with someone that work there. There was a time when this nurse from the hospital went to Haiti and at a wedding, they were playing all the video of people who were in the wedding. She was there watching the video and she said, "Oh! I know her. She's my patient." And they know where she is working and right there and then, people were looking at the video already classifying my friend, not knowing anything. They already give her [an HIV-positive] status, and some of them never met her.

Mona leveraged her status at the hospital in numerous ways, often negotiating for a host of resources for herself and other Haitian clients and navigating issues of confidentiality and needs unrelated to health. During a weekly educational class, for example, a pharmaceutical representative walked into the room while Jaime Silva, the patient educator, was in the middle of a lecture on preventing HIV/AIDS.[3] Jaime stopped his lecture and greeted the representative warmly, as she pulled out some pamphlets. The representative introduced herself and said, as if reading from a brochure: "Kaletra is very easy for patients to take, and they take a round pill twice a day. Individuals that start on Kaletra as their first treatment can take it for four years as a single dose therapy. In our seven-year data, it was found that if a patient takes Kaletra as their first regimen, the majority of them have undetectable viral loads. It's been also shown that their CD4 count has gone up tremendously for patients who take Kaletra as their first regimen." She then pulled out an informational sheet, along with an invitation to a public lecture on "Understanding HIV Resistance" sponsored by Abbott Laboratories and held at a well-known local Cuban steakhouse. Without mentioning Kaletra, Jaime praised the featured speaker and the quality of the restaurant.

Mona quickly offered to be a liaison, suggesting that she could increase Haitian attendance at the lecture. "But transportation might be a barrier . . . could you get us a van?" she added. The representative looked surprised, as if she had not considered the fact that transportation might be a challenge for these clients. She replied: "Although Abbott cannot offer transportation, maybe you could petition Medicaid or the hospital to hire a van for you." "How many people do you need?" asked Mona, without skipping a beat. She wanted to convey her authority to gather a mass of people. She also wanted to gauge how many people would be able to receive food. "What do you mean? The restaurant can accommodate 100 people," the Abbott representative replied, sounding confused. "No, no. She can get people to come," interjected Jaime. The representative nodded, as if she finally understood: "Wow! That's great! Maybe you can get some people and help translate at the dinner. They have a great salad bar, and then they also come to your table and hand-carve meat for you." Mona translated the conversation to the rest of the class. They expressed excitement about free food, even though many knew that they could not attend without free transportation. The representative whispered to Jaime that if Mona could get people to come, "We could figure out something for her." Jaime proudly responded: "Yes, she's really good!"

Mona's influence over other clients both in and out of clinical settings gave her considerable ability to traverse multiple levels of administrative, political, and social activities. Like Jacques and Irene, she epitomizes living positively as the enterprising biocitizen who actively shapes her life through choices based on her biological affliction. However, the example of the Abbott Laboratories event, like that of the opening vignette in this chapter, reveals how the rhetoric of positive living as a form of biological citizenship erases the underlying issues related to the precarious lives of Haitians in Miami. Stories like those of Irene, Mona, and Jacques demonstrate fidelity to certain aspects of positive living and biological citizenship. They also illustrate how the concepts of positive living and biological citizenship can reinforce and advance unequal citizenship by effectively overlooking Haitians' daily struggles with hunger, poverty, lack of adequate safety nets, and routine targeting by biomedical interventions.

Many scholars have maintained that contemporary biological citizenship is markedly different from older notions of citizenship because it is no longer based on racial and sexual biopolitics. Rose and Novas state:

> Inevitably, in discussing these issues, the spectre of racialized national politics, eugenics and racial hygiene is summoned from its sleep. Such biological understanding of human beings [is] clearly related to notions of citizenship and projects of citizen building both at the level of the individual and of the nation-state. Nonetheless, contemporary biological citizenship does not, in the main, take this racialized and nationalised form. The links of biology and human worth and human defects today differ significantly from those of the eugenic age. Different ideas about the role of biology in human worth are entailed in practices of selective abortion, pre-implantation genetic diagnosis and embryo selection. Different ideas about the biological responsibilities of the citizen are embodied in contemporary norms of health and practices of health education. Different citizenship practices can be seen in the increasing importance of corporeality to practices of identity, and in new technologies which intervene upon the body at levels ranging from the superficial (cosmetic surgery) to the molecular (gene therapy). . . . And while it is true that many states are once more regarding the specific hereditary stock of their population as a resource to be managed, these endeavours are not driven by a search for racial purity. Instead, they are grounded in the hope that certain specific characteristics of the genes of groups of their citizens may potentially provide a valuable resource for the generation of intellectual property rights, for biotechnological innovation and the creation of what we will term, following Catherine Waldby, *biovalue.* (2005, 440–41)

I contend that although differences have arisen in how the biological values of populations are managed and conceptualized, citizenship in the West is still exclusionary. As I have shown, for Haitians in Miami, including those like Jacques and Mona who are hailed as models of positive living, HIV/AIDS represents not only a way to garner much-needed resources but also a continuing legacy of unequal citizenship, steeped in various forms of race- and risk-based national identity politics.

As a result of persistent depictions of Haitians as natural carriers of disease,[4] many Haitians continue to distance themselves from biologic associations. That is, many try to secure civil, social, and political rights by detaching any biological attributes from their sense of self and community. This process of removal and separation happens in a number of ways. I discussed some of these issues in the previous section about adherence, disclosure, and safe sex, showing how Haitians have shifted positive living away from its biological underpinnings of disease.

Another way that Haitians decouple notions of biology from the sense of self is through the reimagination of HIV/AIDS as an outcome of multiple effects and as an everyday occurrence of suffering, rather than an exceptional event. For instance, Michelle Dupuy, an older woman who came to class infrequently, often positioned HIV/AIDS as a combination of biomedical conditions and possession by malicious spirits. Michelle invoked these multiple notions of HIV/AIDS during and outside of class. In one Kreyòl clinical class, she argued: "I don't take disease from no man. A woman live with my husband. She wanted to get even with me. She got *juju* [a spell as a result of witchcraft or magic] and sent it to me. She told me to my face that I had to leave my husband or else someone was going to give me HIV virus." Michelle incorporates notions of "disease" and "HIV virus" into a framework that presents jealous others and angry spirits as sources of affliction. Jaime Silva, the non-Haitian educator, asked: "Is it documented that you got it from no man?" The other class members became visibly uncomfortable, with some averting their eyes from Michelle, while others sucked their teeth or whispered to their neighbors. Mona and some of the other clients, fearful that Haitians as a group would once again be marked as ignorant and backward through the rubric of cultural reasoning, forced Jaime to change the subject by saying to him "Do you really want to go there? We don't want you to go there!" The women's reluctance to talk about spiritual affliction was not because they agreed or disagreed with Michelle's position; rather, because of the reaction of Jaime, a non-Haitian provider, they feared confirming the stereotypes that contribute to their continued marginalization and they consciously suppressed any evidence of their difference.

In contrast to Michelle, Renée and others depict HIV/AIDS as nothing out of the ordinary and part of a broader notion of uncontrollable fate. Renée Mevs, a regular at the clinical classes, presented a viewpoint that I would often hear expressed: "For me, HIV is like any other disease. God will eventually take us all, so what is the big deal? Don't we Haitians all suffer in disease and in wellness? It doesn't bother me, because I have a lot more things to worry about than this." For Renée, as for many Haitians, HIV/AIDS is not an extraordinary life event but only one element in a larger cycle of life and death determined solely by God or some other higher power. HIV/AIDS also represents just a fragment of the much larger condition of daily suffering caused by economic, political, and social marginalization. As the anthropologists Paul Farmer (1992) and Karen Brown (1991) have shown, narratives of illness, disease, and suffering often detach human agency from affliction. Brown writes:

> "*Moun fèt pou mouri* [People are born to die]," Haitians are fond of saying, usually with a casual shrug of the shoulders. This proverb gives voice to both the pain of life in poverty-stricken Haiti and the stoic acceptance that, on one level at least, characterizes the Haitian attitude towards this life. *Mizè* (suffering, and, more precisely, the suffering of poverty) is an expected and recurrent condition. . . . Because, for the great majority of Haitians, it is a given that life is filled with struggle and suffering, it is not inaccurate to say that problem-free periods are pervaded with an anxiety that anticipates crises just around the corner. (1991, 345)

The use of Brown's analysis here is not to present Haitians as incapable of understanding and using biomedical models of disease or to reaffirm an explanatory model approach (Young 1982), where the dichotomy is between disease as an organic, natural category and illness as the social and cultural construction of patients' disease. In addition, it is not to say that Renée, Michelle, and others are simply recasting the causes of HIV/AIDS and other misfortunes in terms of local sorcery or supernatural intervention from a need to impute agency. Instead, I argue that their stories serve to dissociate them (and other Haitians) from the solely biological characteristics of HIV/AIDS, which are stressed in the official rhetoric of HIV/AIDS programming. By reconfiguring HIV/AIDS through notions of the continuous susceptibility to suffering as well as through human and spiritual mediations, these Haitians see the biological as simultaneously something that is manipulable and as immutable destiny. These conceptualizations and actions act as a powerful trope that contrasts with the promise of the positive living movement, and they do not function in a space where the biological is knowable and controllable and where acceptance of and despair about an uncertain future are condemned.

Finally, Haitians also strive to dissociate biological configurations of subjectivity and citizenship by not participating in HIV/AIDS prevention. As I discussed in detail in chapters 2 and 3, Haitians rarely participate in clinical and nonclinical HIV prevention programs, compared to other ethnic groups. HIV/AIDS prevention programs at large hospitals like Miami General and other smaller venues, along with provider trainings at the Miami-Dade Department of Health, frequently had to cancel trainings, classes, and programs conducted in Kreyòl due to a lack of participation.[5]

Citizenship by Any Other Name

By focusing on individuals—like Jacques Chantal—who are well-versed in the self-management of risk and garnering resources as a result of their HIV/AIDS affliction, providers and programs promote the notion of positive living without acknowledging the severe economic, political, and social struggles that plague those same individuals. Instead, they instruct clients to be responsible to themselves as well as various others through biosocial practices such as adherence, disclosure, safe sex, advocacy, and activism.

The concepts and strategies of positive living are those of contemporary biological citizenship. However, the notions of biosociality and biological citizenship as new forms of biomedical communities and activism (Rabinow 1992, 1996; Rose 2007; Rose and Novas 2005)—especially in the field of HIV/AIDS, as documented by Steven Epstein (1996) and others—do not exist in the same ways in the context of Haitians in Miami. Various policies have long conceptualized Haitians as biological citizens, through designations as AIDS carriers (Farmer 1992; Farmer and Kim 1991) and people with tainted blood.[6] As a result of a confluence of factors, Haitians were not shaped by the sense of a shared biological identity or numerical subjectivity, unlike the primarily gay activists documented in Epstein's landmark work (1996). These factors include the biomedical, political, and social classifications that continue to cause a tremendous amount of fear of and discrimination toward the Haitian community (Fairchild and Tynan 1994; Farmer 1992; Nachman 1993); the tendency to self-identify not as Haitians but as other black immigrants or as African Americans, as a reaction to existing negative stereotypes of Haitians (Laguerre 1984, 1998; Nachman 1993; Portes and Stepick 1993; Stepick 1992, 1998; Stepick et al. 2003; Zéphir 1996); and resistance to and suspicion of public health educational and intervention programs (Farmer and Kim 1991).

The discussion of positive living allows us to see that notions of biological citizenship inadequately characterize many Haitians' relations to themselves, others, the nation-state, and various communities of transnational citizens. Current discourses of biological citizenship overvalue the manipulability of life because they are based on certain presuppositions that underestimate the potency of social categories of difference—such as race and nationality—that still play a large role in citizenship discourses in the United States. They also overestimate the agency of the afflicted or potentially afflicted by assuming certain kinds of potential for action that those living in poverty, social exclusion, and political marginalization may not possess.

HIV/AIDS programs in Miami that center on positive living remind us that discussions of biological citizenship must take into consideration the fact that particular individuals and groups, like Haitians in Miami, want and strive to be citizens of a nonbiological kind because they are always already implicated in racialized and nationalized citizenship projects that seek to classify them as inherently pathological, unclean, and disease ridden (Farmer 1992; Farmer and Kim 1991; Nachman 1993). Haitians' claims of citizenship rights, as demonstrated through positive living discourses, still may adopt some aspects of biological and scientific reasoning. However, the main focus of individual and collective struggles for political, economic, and social recognition is on the decoupling of citizenship and biology.

5

Treating the Nation

Health Disparities and the Politics of Difference

During my time in Miami, I worked with a variety of public health professionals who advocated for better health outcomes for Haitians. A majority of these providers supported and diligently championed increasingly compartmentalized programming initiatives that sought to personalize prevention messages according to various social categories of difference such as race, gender, and sexual orientation. Rosi Jacques, a Haitian American prevention provider at the Miami-Dade Department of Health, was one such provider with whom I worked closely in understanding the landscape of HIV/AIDS prevention services for Haitians in Miami. She repeatedly expressed concerns about health initiatives aimed at specific racial and ethnic groups. Her sentiments mirrored those I often heard from other providers working with Haitians:

> Now, imagine that when you go into a population like the Haitian community, you can't just say "OK. This is HIV. This is what it is, this is what it's not" because there are so many other things that need to be taught before you can even you can get to that level.
>
> In order for the people to actually grasp the whole concept of very basic HIV information, there needs to a whole type of work that needs to be done at another level before they're even ready to tackle that information, because remember a lot of Haitians that come here . . . you know, they don't read, they don't write, there's a lot of superstition, you know, so how are you going to then come down and say "Oh, this is just a virus that comes in from secretions" . . . you know—Whoa! What is a virus? What is the difference between a virus and bacteria? What do you mean by secretions? You mean somebody just put roots on their hands . . . you understand?

And even for the person who is literate, there are still some barriers. . . . You cannot blanket the prevention message. You cannot blanket the resources, the literature, the posters, even the [public service announcements] to one population because it [HIV] does not hit one population. Like for example, when we were working on our prevention video, we had to choose. We had to choose what kind of Haitian women we are talking about. Because the issues of the participants in that segment are not necessarily the same issues as the other Haitian woman who comes in, who has a household, who has a husband, who has an education, who speaks English very well, who is not even going to be recognized as a Haitian woman unless she decides to identify herself [as such]. And that other person comes in here with a very heavy accent, does not write, doesn't have a husband, doesn't even have a high school diploma. She is still fighting with immigration. You can't tell me that we're talking to the same people here—we're not talking to the same women, you see.

It should not be on a scale of more at risk and less at risk, because risk has to be reconceptualized. We know that a lot of it has to do with education, with the socioeconomic resources, with immigration status. And people are like, "What does that have to do with HIV? What does it have to do with prevention?" It has everything to do with it. Because people are not going to be as receptive to certain things when there are other underlying issues that are a lot more important to them.

Rosi's arguments demonstrate two divergent approaches to the conceptualization of health disparities within a singular view of HIV/AIDS: one emphasizes measuring the impact of the social environment, psychosocial influences, and biological pathways on disparities in health outcomes among populations; the other focuses on contextual social and structural factors that contribute to health differentials. Rosi describes highly complex issues related to poverty and social capital by using standard categories of social epidemiology such as "education," "socioeconomic resources," and "immigration status"—categories often used to measure and monitor health disparities. She portrays Haitians as passive recipients of official interventions ("receptive to certain things") and hindered by cultural "barriers" such as superstition—and also as people who need individually and culturally tailored education and behavioral interventions.

She also asserts that there are broader social and structural forces that must be taken into consideration in HIV/AIDS prevention, labeling them as "other underlying issues that are a lot more important." In this narrative, Haitians are presented as a population so mired in the social and structural violence of daily life that prevention efforts need to address broader issues of illiteracy, poverty, and immigration. Even the concept of risk cannot be "blanketed" and has to be "reconceptualized" because Haitians cannot be lumped into one uniform group. In this dual framing, intervention and prevention solutions can be targeted toward Haitians, both as individuals and as a community. Prevention initiatives can also operate at the structural level, locating solutions away from individual and community actors.

Rosi situates herself, as do others working with Haitians, as a cultural broker who constructs relevant knowledge about HIV/AIDS prevention and about Haitians. Her role is to mediate communication between the official directives of health disparities and HIV/AIDS prevention programming and a passive and uninformed public. She also sees herself as a cultural insider, helping Haitians overcome their cultural and structural restraints so that they are able to access resources.

Many providers and Haitian clients share Rosi's views that reaching Haitians will be difficult if current HIV/AIDS prevention and intervention programs are not overhauled. In clinical educational classes for Haitians about HIV/AIDS prevention, clients often diverted lectures and discussions away from HIV/AIDS transmission and risk to religion, discrimination, and economic and legal struggles. They expressed their desires to have more informative classes on legal, economic, health, and social services. For instance, during a prevention class, a woman whom we had never seen before came in with Julie Bonami, the Haitian educator. This woman looked nervous, as if Julie had forced her to come, and she stared at the floor, her hands tightly clasped. Mona Blanc, the Haitian patient advocate, was thrilled at having a new face in the class. She pointed to the lady and asked her to introduce herself. "Flore," she said, speaking so quietly that we all leaned in to hear her. When Mona asked her to fill out the sign-in sheet, she refused. After Mona coaxed her to in front of the class, she filled it out, explaining that she did not like coming to classes because she was uncomfortable with anyone knowing her "business." She said that she was also tired of hearing about HIV/AIDS. Mona immediately looked at me sternly and began to ask me to write down what she was going to say carefully, because she wanted me to communicate to "the higher-ups" what Haitians really wanted. She explained:

> What I am going to say they probably won't want to do it, but I always think put the Haitian on the phone, put them on the speaker, so they don't see the face. If they don't see the face, they will come. Or if there is a clinic which says you don't have to speak English, you can speak Kreyòl, you better believe it—you not going to meet any Haitian there.
>
> Give Haitians a choice; those who don't want to meet face to face will come to that clinic just because they know someone will translate for them but they don't have to see nobody.
>
> One thing is the entrance door [starts laughing] is not really outside door. They come in the door, they go inside, they do what they have to

do, and they go out of another door. Waiting room should be like little booths. You come and you go into that booth, and in the hallway, there is some health care workers who manage three booth doors that does not open at the same time.

We will get all of those who don't want to come. We will get all of them to come to [health]care. And guess what? If we have a place like that, you better believe it, other places that don't have a place like that would be in trouble because word of mouth . . . because "Hey, you see this clinic, this is the way they do it. It's a lot of confidentiality." Then you will see, they will be leaving the other place and go to our place.

I know this is crazy, but this is the only way you going to get Haitians to come for anything that says HIV. It would be better if you have a clinic that gives everything to you, spiritual, immigration, lawyers, and doctors. But that is not going to happen, so this is the only thing that I think will work for HIV.

Mona responds to Flore's weariness of discussions about HIV/AIDS and discomfort with others' associating her with HIV/AIDS by putting forth what she thinks needs to be done in order to have Haitians participate in such settings. Her plans for HIV/AIDS prevention and treatment sites are elaborately constructed, and she describes measures to ensure that they would provide physical and informational confidentiality. She admits that it would be more beneficial to have a site offering healthcare services as well as legal, spiritual, and other social services, but since "that is not going to happen," having draconian measures to ensure strict confidentiality is the only other alternative.

Rosi and Mona's arguments are rooted in the premise that Haitians are fundamentally different on the basis of being Haitian, a difference that is characterized by superstition, limited education, fear, and ignorance and rooted in race, nationality, and culture. Rosi and Mona advocate for health interventions that include specifically tailored efforts that address these issues of difference because they think that otherwise Haitians will not participate. As they both argue, issues of confidentiality and privacy play a central role in the design of successful HIV/AIDS programs, and lumping all Haitians into a single program fails because there are many differences (for example, in terms of literacy, income, and immigration status) that separate Haitians from each other. In the women's narratives, the notion of difference and disparity comes to stand in for Haitians without a reference group. Haitians are different or have certain disparities in health because of who they inherently are, not necessarily in comparison to another group. These so-called differences in the nature of Haitians—people seen as ignorant, uneducated, and ruled by superstition and fear—become positioned as innate qualities and serve as acceptable ways to understand Haitians and the disparities in their health outcomes.

What Difference Does Difference Make?

In the preceding chapters, I have examined how the growing significance of quantification, the increasing focus on communities and their cultures as the site of risk, and the mounting emphasis on personal empowerment and transformation through illness-based identities in HIV/AIDS programs have all shaped and sustained notions of difference across groups of people. In this chapter, I am interested in how programs organized specifically for racial and ethnic groups have become a normal and natural part of the HIV/AIDS landscape in Miami. In particular, I explore why among providers like Rosi and Mona, policy makers, and the general public there is an overwhelming sense that health disparities in HIV/AIDS must be overcome and that disease interventions and programming intended for specific racial and ethnic groups are fundamental to the success of public health prevention in HIV/AIDS.

In Miami there is an abundance of racially and ethnically based HIV/AIDS intervention initiatives and prevention programs, whose goal is to respond to the severe disparities in transmission and health outcomes among racial and ethnic minority populations. Many of those involved in HIV/AIDS programming, like Rosi and Mona, continually advocate for stratifying programs according to categories of social difference such as race, ethnicity, risk groupings, culture, and nationality. Through surveillance and categorization practices, a new focus on communities as intervention sites, and foundational tenets like positive living, HIV/AIDS programs uphold and reinforce racial and ethnic differences. These categories of difference critically shape the ways HIV/AIDS interventions are administered and understood. Although the use of race and ethnicity in health research continues to be highly debated and problematic among public health researchers and practitioners, in HIV/AIDS programs, "race" and "ethnicity" encompass multiple meanings, represent a confluence of biological and social factors, and heavily influence research and policy decisions.[1] Concepts of race and ethnicity are foundational to the understanding of health disparities and are fundamentally entwined in the discourses and practices of HIV/AIDS prevention in the United States.

In this chapter, I first explore how racial and ethnic differences, particularly in HIV/AIDS-related health outcomes, have come to be naturalized as common facts that no longer need to be explained or deliberated. In particular, I am interested in what it means to naturalize health disparities, why it matters, and what the implications of this naturalization are. Second, I illustrate how the notion of health disparities operates in people's interpretation of HIV/AIDS programs and how Haitians are expected to and do respond to those programs. I am concerned with what these disparities reveal about how providers like Rosi and Mona perceive the relationship between racial and ethnic difference and health outcomes. Whose difference is described within the framework of health disparities? What does this imply? What is assumed about the people who are not targets of HIV/AIDS interventions?

Disparity and differences are relational terms in public health and are used to denote variation from the established norm or standard. For instance, if a particular health outcome is seen at a higher or lower rate in a population compared to the norm, it would be considered a disparity between those two groups. Difference also indicates the quality of being not alike, distinct, or different from what is otherwise known. However, notions of disparity and difference, in the field of HIV/AIDS prevention, no longer need to be relational to confer meaning: the terms themselves have come to describe essential and distinguishing attributes of individuals and groups of people, frequently along lines of social difference or risk. In other words, disparity or difference is used and understood to describe Haitians and their poor health outcomes without the mention of a standard reference group for comparison. In this way health disparities have come to be highly influential in the science and practice of public health, controlling material and social resources and making possible various funding, research, and social agendas. By reconceptualizing the realm of health disparities as being exceedingly productive, generative, and valuable to the management and operation of public health, we might begin to make some headway in improving our responses to people's needs for better health care access and outcomes.

Unhealthy People: Framing Health Disparities

The beginning of research and policy interest in the concept of health disparities is difficult to date, but those interests have existed for over a century in various forms. Scholars such as the physician Barbara Starfield (2006) date their history back to Friedrich Engels's *The Condition of the Working-Class in England in 1844* (1950). Engels documents disparities in disease prevalence and outcomes as a result of the Industrial Revolution and argues that the working class was worse off after that revolution due to diseases attributed to occupational hazards and neighborhood living conditions. Since the publication of this classic work, health and social structures have increasingly been linked. In 1948 the United Nations adopted the Universal Declaration of Human Rights, proclaiming that the right to health is fundamental to individual and social existence, forms the basis for global citizenship, and is ensured by other rights and freedoms (Farmer 1999, 2003; Mann et al. 1999). Implicit in this affirmation is the belief that both governments and individuals must play a central role in ensuring that such rights are achieved.

In the United States these broader and complex linkages between social environment and adverse health outcomes have given way to unquestioned associations among notions of race, ethnicity, and health disparities. Due to a historical legacy of slavery and segregation, race and ethnicity have been long considered factors in access to and quality of health care in the United States and have been the driving force of much research and activism around disparities in health (Gamble and Stone 2006). As Rosi's and Mona's narratives demonstrate, race and ethnicity have become the cornerstones of discourses of health disparities, in which linkages among health, human rights, and citizenship have been translated almost exclusively through the concepts of race and ethnicity.

In turn, the elimination of racial and ethnic disparities in health care and outcomes has become a critical role for government. The US Department of Health and Human Services, for example, created the Healthy People initiative in 1980, with a set of goals to be achieved by 1990. The department established national strategies to reduce mortality and chronic disease morbidity by, for example, improving health status, health-related risks, public awareness, surveillance measures, research efforts, and health services. Each following decade brought a new set of goals to be attained and populations to be targeted. Healthy People 2000 differed from the initiative of the preceding decade because set objectives had to be measurable to ensure evidence-based monitoring of progress (National Center for Health Statistics 2001). The objectives for 2000 included language about reducing health disparities for the first time, in the belief that "progress towards a healthier America will depend substantially on improvements for certain populations that are at especially high risk" (US Department of Health and Human Services 1994, 29). The goal was to reduce the gap in health between the population overall and population groups deemed to have increased incidences of morbidity and mortality, including people with low incomes, those from racial and ethnic minority groups, and those with disabilities (see table 5.1).

For 2010 this goal was changed to eliminating health disparities among certain demographic groups, including women and racial and ethnic minorities, using a multidisciplinary approach involving individuals, communities, and national organizations. In the Healthy People 2010 report, disparities in health outcomes were contextualized as the result of convergences of genetic variation, environmental factors, and specific health behaviors; however, most population-based objectives were monitored according to how groups, based on their racial and ethnic differences, measured in comparison to each other (P. Lee et al. 2001; US Department of Health and Human Services 2001). In addition, the scientific evidence that influenced these goals focused on race and ethnicity as categories of natural distinction, which as a result, were used to design the framework for improving health status and largely determined the measures of success needed to achieve such goals (P. Lee et al. 2001).

TABLE 5.1

Evolution of Healthy People 2020

Target Year	1990	2000	2010	2020
Overarching Goals	• Decrease mortality: infants— adults • Increase independence among older adults	• Increase span of healthy life • Reduce health disparities • Achieve access to preventive services for all	• Increase quality and years of healthy life • Eliminate health disparities	• Attain high-quality, longer lives free of preventable disease • Achieve health equity; eliminate disparities • Create social and physical environments that promote good health • Promote quality of life, health development, healthy behaviors across life stages
Topic areas	15	22	28	42[a]
Objectives/ measures	226/n.a.[b]	312/n.a.[b]	467/n.a.[b]	580/1,200

Source: Adapted from US Department of Health and Human Services, "Healthy People 2020" (Washington: US Department of Health and Human Services, 2011; accessed July 22, 2013, http://www.healthypeople.gov/2020/GetInvolved/Healthy PeoplePresentation_2_24_11.ppt).

[a]Healthy People 2020 includes forty-two topic areas, thirty-nine of which have objectives.

[b]Not applicable.

In the Healthy People 2020 report, the focus was on health equity,[2] health disparities,[3] and determinants of health.[4] For 2020 the goals were expanded to "achieve health equity, eliminate disparities, and improve the health of all groups" by focusing on the determinants of health (US Department of Health

and Human Services 2010). However, monitoring and measuring health disparities by race and ethnicity still continues to be a significant focus.

Although discussions about the concept of health disparities are varied and
numerous, there is no broad consensus on how to define such disparities. One
broad definition is that health disparities are the differences, variations, and
inequalities in health outcomes across individuals and groups. The social epidemiologists Olivia Carter-Pokras and Claudia Baquet (2002) argue that there
are at least eleven concepts of health disparities and that the adoption of any
of them would have different repercussions for research and policy. The World
Health Organization defines health inequalities as "composite measures of
the variations in health status across individuals in a population" (Murray et
al. 1999, 537), while US institutions such as the Institute of Medicine and the
Centers for Disease Control and Prevention (CDC) link race and ethnicity to
disparities. The institute calls disparities in health care "racial or ethnic differences in the quality of healthcare that are not due to access-related factors or
clinical needs, preferences, and appropriateness of intervention" (Smedley et al.
2003, 32). The CDC contends that disparities are unequal "burden[s] of illness
and death experienced by blacks or African Americans, Hispanics or Latinos,
American Indians and Alaska Natives, and Native Hawaiian and Other Pacific
Islanders, compared to the U.S. population as a whole. . . . These disparities are
believed to be the result of the complex interaction among genetic variations,
environmental factors, and specific health behaviors" (Centers for Disease Control and Prevention 2007a).

Furthermore, the physician and medical historian Vanessa Gamble and the
political scientist Deborah Stone highlight the differences between the terms
"disparity" and "inequity": "Disparity is a descriptive term that refers to differences between population groups in health status or access to medical care.
It carries no moral loading and no connotation of right or wrong. Inequity is a
normative term. Inherent in its meaning is a critique of differences as unfair,
unjust, or morally wrong. The choice of terms is a matter of political strategy as
well as meaning" (2006, 96). Although choosing one term instead of the other
may have to do with "political strategy as well as meaning," in the field of HIV/
AIDS the two terms are used interchangeably. The term "disparity," for instance,
has come to be intrinsically both descriptive and normative in meaning. In the
above definitions by the Institute of Medicine and the CDC, "disparity" indicates phenomena that are not only inherently linked to race and ethnicity but
also result from the interplay among social and physical environments, individual behaviors, and genetic factors. "Disparity" is not merely descriptive; it
implies that a set of phenomena have a negative value, and thus the differences
constituting the disparity need to be acted on—that is, reduced and eventually
eliminated—and managed in the name of morality, ethics, and human rights.

Approaches to Health Disparities

There are two major approaches to health disparities in the current literature. The first is reflected in a series of studies that are rooted in social epidemiological thought and positivist methodologies and are devoted to establishing the chain of disease risk causation from the social environment, psychosocial influences, and biological pathways. These studies are varied and complex, and—much like Rosi's arguments about education levels and immigration status being risk factors for HIV/AIDS—they naturalize structural and social inequality by first reducing broader forces and identities such as socioeconomic characteristics, race, ethnicity, and gender into calculable variables, and then accepting these variables as fundamental causes of disparities in health status. Some of the studies focus on life-course approaches to explain health inequalities, tracing how hazardous exposures affect the body from before birth until death and the ways in which risk accumulates or is refracted through critical periods of exposure (Wadsworth 1997). Others, like the Epidemiological Catchment Area Study,[5] highlight broader social determinants such as stress and various psychosocial factors to clarify the workings of health inequalities. There is also a body of work that discusses the complex relations between income inequality, social capital, and population health. For instance, Eugene Rogot and colleagues (1992) analyzed data from the National Longitudinal Mortality Study and concluded that people with higher incomes and more education have a lower risk of mortality than those with lower incomes and less education. Still others argue that there are gradients in health outcomes that are continuous across the socioeconomic spectrum and that therefore cannot be "due to absolute material standards" (G. Smith 2003, xxxiv). The Whitehall Study, conducted by Michael Marmot and his colleagues (1987), revealed that British civil servants, who were considered neither the richest nor the poorest in society, had a social gradient of health and disease. That is, the lower an individual was in the "social" hierarchy, the higher her or his risk of disease. Marmot and his coauthors (1987) claimed that even when they controlled for unhealthy behaviors such as smoking, drinking, and a sedentary lifestyle—which could have been the consequences of an individual's position in the social hierarchy—the evidence pointed to more direct pathways to explain stratification and health. In other words, the inequalities attributed to income or wealth or lifestyle factors were important but not sufficient to account entirely for risk of disease; a person who was higher on the socioeconomic gradient was exposed to more environmental and occupational stressors and higher levels of stress, which could have physiological and psychosocial effects, greatly increasing the person's risk of disease.

Although these studies focus on complex and interdependent relations contributing to social stratification, they tend to condense these factors into quantifiable variables and measures such as socioeconomic status (SES) or social capital. The variables then take on a life of their own, so that the notion that SES is no longer seen as a total measure of various complex economic and social factors such income, education, occupation, work experience, and economic and social position. Variables such as SES become divorced from the intricate web of relations that make up the social structures from which they were derived and become representative of risk itself. Risk is directly mapped onto these variables, so that SES—instead of the individual or collective social and economic factors that have been combined to form SES—becomes a risk factor for poor health outcomes. The social history and the process of constructing these variables become invisible, and variables such as SES come to be seen as real and actual representations of complex processes.

Much in the same way, risk also becomes a material reality. The inherent assumption is that the components (such as SES, race, ethnicity, and income) underlying risk exist universally, as do the mechanisms—intervention and treatment—used to reduce risk. This way of viewing and positioning risk makes it possible for formal scientific analyses of risk to render it and the factors that are said to contribute to it universal, common, and easily measurable. As a result, intervention, treatment, and prevention efforts for risk reduction focus on prevention measures such as individual- and community-level education and behavioral change. Even though enumerative descriptions at the level of groups and populations (assessing SES, income, and social capital, for example) do not necessarily pertain to the individuals within a given group,[6] programs focusing on individual-level behavior change and education are seen as indisputably beneficial and well understood and are said to be well received by those at risk.

The other major approach to health disparities originates in the social sciences, from a neo-Marxist political economy of health framework (Baer et al. 1997; Bourgois 2003; Farmer 1999, 2003; Navarro 2000, 2004; Singer 1998). This approach has been taken up more recently by public health researchers who focus on the relationship between social determinants and population health outcomes and risk for disease (Commission on Social Determinants of Health 2008; Raphael 2006). They argue that the economic, social, and political power of transnational governmental, nongovernmental, and industrial establishments increasingly leads to policies that shifted focus from labor to capital, deregulated labor markets, and decelerated redistribution through the welfare state—all of which widened social inequalities in health. This kind of framing begins with the understanding that lived experiences of individuals and groups are embedded in a complex web of history, social status, power, structural context, and culture. As a result, broader social and structural forces need to be evaluated more critically in epidemiological and public health analyses, replacing existing reductionist and cursory models of factors contributing to risk.

The physician and anthropologist Paul Farmer, one of the most influential proponents of this model, addresses these issues in a compelling piece about the Haitian poor. He and Didi Bertrand (2000) write that poor health in Haiti is attributable not to causes within the country—poverty and ecology—as claimed by policy makers and public health officials, but to transnational forces outside of the country—slavery, colonialism, forced isolation, despotic rule, military occupation, political instability, and structural development programs. These adverse and deeply rooted processes have given rise to conditions that led to the poor health and limited well-being of the majority of Haitians. Farmer and Bertrand argue that "social forces—that is, historically given economic and cultural forces—determine, to a large extent, the health of the Haitian people. . . . One of Haiti's lessons for social medicine is that social conditions will to a large extent determine patterns of morbidity and mortality, and that the strength of this association is amplified as conditions worsen. That is, the health *sequelae* of structural violence are most severe among the poor. Unfortunately, epidemiology and public health are increasingly uninterested in such broad analyses" (2000, 87–88). Many social scientists similarly advocate for approaches that link local contexts to larger geopolitical processes. Rather than reject biological, psychological, and epidemiological approaches to the study of social phenomena, anthropologists and other social scientists—as well as a growing body of public health researchers—promote critical studies of complex biosocial interactions among environment, history, and culture (Nguyen and Peschard 2003).

In this approach, biomedically and epidemiologically focused discourses of risk are seen as contributing to the "desocialization" of poor health (Farmer et al. 1996, 198), and the ontological relations between risk and health disparities are constructed as oppositional. Health disparities are seen as concrete and natural because they result from broader shifts in economic, social, and political environments, while risk is conceptualized as a component of the subjective and value-laden rationality of individuals and institutions. For instance, in a scathing criticism of dominant public health literature focusing on poor women and HIV/AIDS, Joe Rhatigan and colleagues (1996) posit that the majority of epidemiological studies of risk not only fail to thoroughly examine multiple associations among gender inequality, poverty, and HIV/AIDS but also locates risk at the level of the individual, divorcing risk from larger social and structural constructs. Risk, in this approach, is seen as embedded in epistemological trends of epidemiology and public health and operates through broader formations of structural violence. The production of the rationalities of risk itself—discourses, assessments, and categories—emanates from combinations of technical, sociocultural, economic, and institutional factors, arrangements through which risk becomes real and accessible to intervention (see Nguyen and Peschard 2003). According to such perspectives, solutions to health disparities are located away from individual actors and communities in more sociologically and culturally informed analyses of the complex relations between health inequalities and the social and structural conditions that create, stabilize, and propagate them.

These two approaches to health disparities represent two very different strands of scholarship, but their frameworks—one based in epidemiological and positivist considerations and the other in the political economy of health—often merge in grounded practice through local initiatives and serve to increasingly naturalize racial and ethnic disparities in health. Providers like Rosi and Mona, for instance, frequently blend both perspectives in their narratives and in their provision of HIV/AIDS prevention programming. They support improving the health standards of Haitians through educational initiatives, behavioral interventions, and other prevention measures. They also advocate for broader social and structural changes to improve the overall living conditions of their Haitian clients. But the underlying foundation of their argument, similar to those of the two major approaches to health disparities, is one that constructs Haitians as fundamentally different from other people and their poor health outcomes as naturally occurring due to their differences. These approaches to health disparities are varied in how they construct groups as different. The first approach, rooted in epidemiology, increasingly compartmentalizes people's social environment so that their SES, social capital, educational level, and income become the basis of their difference and disparity. In the political economy of health approach, difference is constituted through broader global economic, political, and social forces that routinely render some people poor and without good health.

The Productive Space of Health Disparities

The concept of health disparity extends far beyond research and scholarship, reaching into policies, programs, and practices. The reduction of health disparities has become one of the top priorities of the US Department of Health and Human Services, and the department has continually increased its budget to reflect this. In fiscal year 2000 it budgeted $145 million for health disparities initiatives (US Department of Health and Human Services 1999); in fiscal year 2010 its budget included $354 million for such activities (US Department of Health and Human Services 2009). Institution building at the national and local levels has also increased significantly. In 1986 the department established an Office of Minority Health (OMH) to address racial and ethnic disparities in health in response to the 1985 report of the Secretary's Task Force on Black and Minority Health (US Department of Health and Human Services 1985). OMH's primary mission is to coordinate agency-wide efforts in improving "the health of racial and ethnic minority populations through the development of health policies and programs that will help eliminate health disparities" (US Department of Health and Human Services 2011a). This office was reauthorized through the Patient Protection and Affordable Care Act of 2010, and the six agencies under Department of Health and Human Services, including the CDC, were required to establish their own offices of minority health. The CDC has had such an office since 1988; its goal has been to "promote health and quality of life by preventing and controlling the disproportionate burden of disease, injury and disability among racial and ethnic minority populations" (Centers for Disease Control and Prevention 2005). In September 2005 the CDC transformed its Office of Minority Health into the Office of Minority Health and Health Disparities. The new office expanded on the goal of its predecessor by having "a broader focus on reducing health disparities experienced by populations defined by race/ethnicity, socio-economic status, geography, gender, age, disability status, and risk status related to sex and gender" (Centers for Disease Control and Prevention 2007a). In 2011 the office was realigned and again received a new name: the Office of Minority Health and Health Equity, whose goal is "to accelerate CDC's health impact in the U.S. population and to eliminate health disparities for vulnerable populations as defined by race/ethnicity, socio-economic status, geography, gender, age, disability status, risk status related to sex and gender, and among other populations identified as at-risk for health disparities" (Centers for Disease Control and Prevention 2012).

Because of two implicit assumptions involved, it is important to consider these changes in the function of the office, from "promot[ing] health and quality of life" for racial and ethnic minorities to "reducing health disparities" and to "eliminat[ing] health disparities" for populations at risk for health disparities. The first assumption is that populations seen to be susceptible for health disparities have expanded from racial and ethnic minorities ("minority health") to a variety of groups seen to be at risk ("minority health and health disparities"). The term "health disparities" became part of official institutional titles around 2005, and the semantic shift from health promotion ("promot[ing] health and quality of life") to the prevention and control of health disparities (reducing or eliminating them) indicates that the disproportionate burden of disease is no longer being left to probability; that anticipatory preventive action against this occurrence is no longer possible; and the only possibilities of intervention, reduction and elimination, must occur reactively.

The gradual semantic move that increasingly conceptualizes health disparities as reducible and eliminable reinforces the notions that the disparities are tangible and naturally occurring and that they are firmly entrenched in our society. Notions of reduction and elimination also suggest that there are acceptable levels of difference among population groups that can now be measured to monitor progress through national objectives such as the Healthy People initiatives. Both the material reality of health disparities and the enumeration of difference help shape how the notions of disparity and difference are understood, received, and given meaning by the very people they are assumed to describe and those who act on them as experts.

Difference and disparity become reduced to discourses of health outcomes, their impacts, and the practices of reducing and eliminating them. The complex social histories and the processes involved in the construction of these differences (such as surveillance practices, a programmatic focus on communities, and an emphasis on illness-based identities) are left untouched and made invisible, so that notions of difference and disparity can stand alone as essential attributes without necessarily implying a relationship between two groups. For instance, the CDC's Office of Minority Health and Health Equity's "vulnerable" and "at-risk" populations represent groups that are seen as inherently different, without any mention of whom they are being compared to (the reference group). The implicit assumption is that there are invulnerable groups that are not at risk, but who are they and how they came to be invulnerable no longer need to be mentioned or cited in order for difference or disparity (through notions of vulnerability and risk) to be seen and have meaning.

Health disparities, in this sense, have come to exist in the realm of the factual and measurable, where their existence is no longer debatable or questionable. As Bruno Latour (1987; Latour and Woolgar 1986) argues, facts arise when there is no longer deliberation about something of which we have come to be convinced, and when the various processes central to such successful persuasion become obsolete. He compares facts to the cybernetician's black box, which represents something whose structure and composition becomes taken for granted. In his discussion of BilDil, the "race-specific" drug for heart failure, Jonathan Kahn has shown that many of these "facts" behind health disparities no longer need proper citations or any citations at all because they have "entered the commonsense realm of accepted reality" (2003, 475).

Similarly, health variations among populations such as the differential rates of HIV/AIDS among racial and ethnic groups in Miami-Dade County no longer need to be explained, for they have come to illustrate an authoritative truth about reality. We no longer need to contemplate the existence of health disparities in HIV/AIDS. Even the vast outpouring of numbers and statistics that are used to bolster claims of the existence of health disparities do not need or require any explanation or clarification. The idea of predisposition to disease through biological, environmental, and social factors becomes innately entangled with the concepts of race and ethnicity. Disparities in health and, in turn, difference situated along racial and ethnic lines have come to be seen as endemic in society. Notions of race and ethnicity are now inherently characteristic of disparities in health and serve to justify the construction and management of programmatic solutions based solely on race and ethnicity. Race, ethnicity, and health disparities have become natural bedfellows; their linkages are increasingly solidified and their authority expands through the very nature of their associations.

Disparities as Matters of Life and Death

This black-boxing of health disparities and differences matters because of the implications it holds for people like the Haitians in Miami. Much like the two approaches to health disparities described above, there is an overwhelming sense in that in health research, tabulations of vulnerabilities to disease specific to racial and ethnic groups are fundamental to the success of public health prevention in HIV/AIDS (Marcelin and Marcelin 2001; Martin et al. 1995; Needle et al. 2003). Advocates of this perspective align themselves with HIV/AIDS literature demonstrating that the epidemic is taking root deeply in impoverished and marginalized communities, where underlying issues pertaining to broader sociopolitical and economic factors serve as driving forces of the epidemic (Farmer 1992; Levenson 2004; Scheper-Hughes 1994; Singer 1998; Sobo 1995). Many health advocates and practitioners in Miami, like Rosi and Mona, promote individual-level educational and behavioral prevention measures while also arguing for the development of programs that address unequal, inadequate, or inaccessible services; educational and employment vacuums; structural underdevelopment and dependency; racism; sexism; and homophobia, along with HIV/AIDS prevention.

Many providers and clients in Miami view HIV/AIDS prevention programs targeted specifically at certain racial and ethnic minorities as beneficial and necessary. Dr. Jones, a prominent physician who runs a hospital clinic that serves only HIV-positive Haitians in Miami, declared: "I think that these programs are helping minorities and people of color because, if not for these programs, they'd be in big trouble. So despite all the misgivings and the inadequacies, thank God that they are there because without them, they'd [the people would] be gone! So . . . thank God for all these things we have." In spite of his "misgivings" about HIV/AIDS prevention programs specifically designed for "minorities" and "people of color," Jones believed that these groups of people would be "in big trouble" or "gone" without such programs. There are two assumptions here: first, that these programs are literally keeping racial and ethnic minority populations alive; and second, that the programs reinforce the notion of the fundamental differences of these groups, while leaving unquestioned the categories of people serving as reference groups from which they are supposedly deviating. Dr. Jones's assertion that prevention programs represent matters of life and death for certain groups of people exemplifies the ways in which both epidemics and the responses to them continue to be mediated through notions of difference in absolute terms.

This narrative of the life-saving benefits of HIV/AIDS programs targeted at minorities is one that I heard often, even in free clinics that were continually struggling for funds and resources. At Sante Ayisyen, a local health clinic in Little Haiti, both Jasmine Desmaret, an HIV/AIDS case manager, and Jerome Meus, an HIV counselor, felt that prevention programs geared toward minority populations were working very well because they were seeing more people in the clinic than ever before. Jasmine explained: "Years ago, we used to have to hunt to basically get ten people to test. Now, we're telling people to come back because so many people are coming to get tested. People are coming on their own to get their results without [our] even having to call them. So I think that the word is getting out that it's OK to get tested, it's OK to know, it's fine, you have to know how to protect yourself. I think it's good because you see kids now are coming to get condoms. They're like 'Hmmm . . . I'm not going in there if I'm not having a condom. I'm not having sex without a condom.' So it's a positive thing." Jasmine reasoned that more people coming into clinics to get tested and to receive basic preventive health services signaled success. This achievement is attributed to the uptake of educational and behavioral interventions such as testing and condom initiatives.

Other providers said that if these racially and ethnically based programs were not working, statistics would "show" disproportionate rises in HIV/AIDS rates in certain groups for whom such programs are designed and targeted. When I showed these informants materials from the Florida Department of Health that highlighted the disproportionate rates of HIV/AIDS in Miami-Dade County and in Florida overall for minority populations, they did not fault the programs directly. Having both internalized the hegemony of enumeration and accepted the ecological fallacy whereby group-level indications of a rise in HIV/AIDS rates are assumed to apply at the level of individuals as well, they felt that this was a problem of "uptake": the people who were the targets of interventions failed to understand and change their risky behavior. Greg Vieux, an HIV counselor at a community-based clinic, for example, told me:

> I don't think there is much I would have to change [about minority-targeted prevention programs]. I believe everything that has been designed works. Look at the gay and lesbian community; they are very knowledgeable about the disease, and there is a big decrease in that community. It's only in the black community that the disease is increasing. So definitely something is going on there. Like I said, I don't believe that they don't get the information; the information is accessible. Now what they do with that information once they get it is a different thing. Why is it that the information is available to everybody and everybody knows it, and the disease is still going up in black communities?

Although he did not explicitly state why he thought the rates were increasing among blacks, Greg clearly believes that the root causes were not at the programmatic level. His statement that "what they do with that information once they get it is a different thing" clearly puts the burden of responsibility on, and tacitly blames, black communities. It is their implied difference from the "gay and lesbian community," used here as a reference group, that makes them susceptible to higher rates of HIV/AIDS. In enumerative practices of calculating health disparities, groups based on sexual identity (such as gays and lesbians) would not typically serve as a reference group for those categorized by race and ethnicity because to do so would be seen as measuring different things (sexual identity versus racial or ethnic identity).[7] Greg constructed difference as that between those who were "knowledgeable about the disease" and those who were not using the information being given to decrease their susceptibility to HIV/AIDS. In practice, the notion of difference or disparity is often constructed as nonrelational, as an essential or distinguishing attribute of someone; and when reference groups are used, they often do not match comparable epidemiological categories (for example, black communities versus gay and lesbian communities).

Even providers who worked closely with Haitian clients told me that institutions were doing a good job of testing people and getting the information out about prevention and intervention. They reasoned that Haitians were not doing "everything [programs] educate them to do because they do whatever they want to do." Jaime Silva, one of the most passionate and dedicated HIV/AIDS prevention educators whom I met during my fieldwork, repeatedly warned me about "giving [Haitians] too much credit." He was well versed in multiple approaches to conducting HIV/AIDS prevention education targeting Haitians, was very respected by all of his Haitian clients, and was openly HIV-positive himself. During our frequent conversations about my research, he would listen empathetically, nodding frequently to demonstrate that he understood my arguments, only to turn around and lecture me gently. "Yes, I understand, but it's really about education," he would say patiently. "These people have almost no level of education. I mean I can see some of them who are learning and who are interested, but most of them. . . . it's nothing. They are just not listening . . . they are not getting it at all. We have to do something, try to really educate, get them to understand certain concepts about the disease." Like Rosi in the opening vignette of this chapter, Dr. Jones, and other providers mentioned above, Jaime considers Haitians to be what Charles Briggs and Daniel Hallin term "biocommunicable outsiders," people who "fail even to acquire the knowledge that would permit them to fashion themselves as biological citizens" (2007, 50–51). Through providers like these, dominant frameworks of public health prevention in HIV/AIDS discursively deny Haitians any form of neoliberal subjectivity—a chance to play the role of responsible consumers who actively manage their health and risk of disease—by portraying them as inherently different, having "no level of education" or interest, and being kept alive by HIV/AIDS programs (see also Briggs and Hallin 2007; Clarke et al. 2003; Rose 2007).

These same providers also marked Haitians as different because of their structural impediments. These barriers made it nearly impossible for the providers to effectively translate and disseminate information to their clients. Many felt that these differences helped to widen the divergences between public health preventives and Haitians. For instance, Jasmine from Sante Ayisyen recounted how disconnected her clients were from the HIV/AIDS programs that target them:

> I went to a training for case managers, and they told me that when a client comes in, have the client to give you a proof of their financial documents, go through their financial screening, and have them write a letter saying that they are the person supporting themselves. But 90 percent of the people that I deal with don't even know how to read and write. And they tell you that you cannot write the letter for them. You know, it's like when you're in a meeting, you are the only one that's dealing with the vast majority of minorities, and I'm like, "this is bullshit." I write the letter for them and tell them what the letter says, and now it's up to them to get it notarized. A lot of them decline my help to send them to English classes. Why? Because they can't go to school because they have to go to the farm or they have to do an odd job, they have to take care of the kids, or if their families send for them, they're taking care of the kids of the family. They're being basically treated like slaves in the house, and they're probably sleeping in a room somewhere. They don't have money to catch a bus; there's not enough bus passes. . . . I only get six bus passes a month and I have to give it to the handicapped, the blind, the incoherent person, you know. What can you do? It's a lose-lose situation.

Like those who advocate political-economy-of-health approaches to health disparities, this case manager describes vividly the practices and assumptions of HIV/AIDS prevention programs that—through the portrayal of Haitians as perpetually uneducated, impoverished, and enslaved—keep structural violence intact and prevent Haitian clients from accessing the safety nets supposedly available to them. She frames her own position as one betwixt and between—"helping" clients access services through unofficial improvisation, while lamenting case management protocols that fail to address the structural constraints of clients with financial and literacy barriers. Jasmine simultaneously questions and reinscribes the potency of difference that frames the portrayal of Haitians.

Even at the county health department, there were parallel opinions about the constraints of HIV/AIDS prevention programs focused on minority groups. For instance, Geri Rodriguez, an HIV/AIDS prevention manager, said:

> When we were doing education and outreach back in the mid-1990s, one of our priority groups was in Little Havana. The prevention wasn't successful, and we were really having a hard time getting through or getting people enrolled. We did a community needs assessment, and we had come up with ten critical priorities of the community. These included gang violence, lack of work, immigration—and health was number five. So we convened a town hall meeting and we got the chief of police to talk about the gang violence, we got an immigration lawyer to talk about immigration issues. People really felt like we listened. They felt respected. We need to start listening again because it was working. We need to understand that behavior is a function of personal situation. The way that we do things now is to aggregate data points about clients, and the politicians want answers to see if behaviors are changing. This is the problem with public health; we don't have time or the money to really find out what is going on.

Geri's attitude reflects her dissatisfaction with the changes in public health prevention itself, which she believes perpetuates the structural barriers faced by her clients through its formulaic and standardized methods that are governed by evidence-based science and larger political conventions. She challenges public health's aggregative imperative through epidemiology in terms of its determination of prevention measures at the level of groups and populations. She also questions operationalizing public health through health promotion with a focus on local communities. She argues that understanding populations through an on-the-ground approach focused on small-scale communities is a better way to adequately determine public health needs, which means that more personal and sustained interactions with community members facilitates the uptake of information and interventions. Her model depicts the community of individuals in Little Havana as active agents who were able to demand certain kinds of resources through nonparticipation, while portraying public health specialists as facilitators that aid the community members in getting what they want and tailor prevention programs toward community needs. For Geri, this process of shifting scales and understanding communities on the ground as opposed to from above is a better way to understand and get at "what is going on."

Fred Dussy—a rural migrant service manager in Florida City and Homestead, areas in which a majority of the population is defined by public health authorities as members of racial or ethnic minority groups—reiterated Geri's sentiments:

I don't like the way that prevention is done now, telling people to practice abstinence or giving them condoms. I think that intervention and
prevention programs were working fine when we had to interact a lot
with people. Like for me, for example, I like to put myself on their level,
like I just dress with a T-shirt and pants, and I talk to them like I would
anybody else. This worked well for immigrants. They are not educated
enough, and that's what we need to do more in immigrant communities. This is true for our population because it's a very rural community,
and it's better to go door to door, to go out there and understand what
is going on instead of just expecting to pass out condoms and have them
come in when they are infected. The whole CDC way of doing things is
more political bullshit than anything else.

Fred sees himself as following a different mode of conducting prevention than
what is mandated by institutional authorities such as the CDC. He claims that by
placing himself on the "level" of his clients—that is, by occupying their (ostensi-
bly outsider) subject position, he can better "understand what is going on." Like
Geri and Jasmine, Fred describes institutional prevention measures by the CDC
as perpetuating rather than alleviating disproportionate rates of disease. He uses
his clients' difference—their rural, immigrant, and uneducated sensibilities—
as evidence to argue against institutional frameworks of HIV/AIDS prevention
and to promote his own alternatives.

Health disparities are perceived and acted on by providers through multiple framings, often mirroring scholarly approaches to health disparities. For
many providers, race and ethnicity are important elements in the provision of
health and health care, and programs aimed at specific racial and ethnic groups
are fundamental to HIV/AIDS prevention. By pathologizing difference, whether
through race, ethnicity, educational level, immigrant status, literacy level, or
social capital, providers support current public health prevention measures targeting individual-level educational and behavioral interventions. At the same
time, they also use difference to expose public health's maintenance of the
structures and practices that perpetuate inequalities in health.

Thinking beyond Difference

Difference continues to become increasingly naturalized at a time when convergences of new and older shifts in politics, economics, biology, medicine, and
technology have opened up complex and multiple sites of transformation for
both humans and nonhumans. In response, building on the work of Michel Foucault's governmentality and biopower theses (1978, 1979, 2003), some scholars
have proclaimed that inequality and stratification are part and parcel of our
postmodern times (Clarke et al. 2003; Dumit 2003; Franklin and Lock 2003;

Lock et al. 2000; Rabinow 1999; Rose 1999, 2007; Thompson 2005). Their framing aligns with David Harvey's work on the paradox of postmodernity, the
simultaneous celebration of fragmentation as well as the embrace of unification
(globalization) in an increasingly transnational and commodity-driven world
(1989). They argue that these recent shifts in science and technology have led to
the selective targeting and exclusion of groups based on race, gender, and class;
they also claim that the shifts themselves are generated by the same stratifying
practices. Stratifications based on race, gender, and class, therefore, give rise to,
are reproduced by, and are co-constitutive of the processes of the larger shifts
in identity and governance.

   This scholarship makes an overlooked but critical contribution to current
approaches of understanding difference and health disparities. These studies,
which stress the recent shifts in focus in health from the diagnosis and treatment
of disease through clinical mediation to risk factor analyses and prevention, are
crucial to the understanding of the increasing importance of surveillance practices and technologies, such as the Program Evaluation and Monitoring System
and the Serological Testing Algorithm for Recent HIV Seroconversions, and con-
sumer- or patient-centered models of HIV/AIDS prevention, such as the "positive living" movement. I use this scholarship to reconfigure health disparities as
a site of authoritative knowledge production about the differential distribution
of disease. I argue that a governmentality framing allows us to focus on the ways
in which health disparities continue to reproduce schemes of hegemony and
structural violence while also attending to the productive capacity of health disparities in determining new forms of citizenship and governance, and that—if
brought into dialogue with current approaches to health disparities—this body
of work might broaden our perspectives.

   Using this scholarship, which builds on studies of governmentality, I
do not directly challenge those who argue that biosocial factors and global-
izing and industrial practices are harmful to a growing number of individuals. Instead, throughout the book and in this chapter, I focus on forms of
knowledge, discourses, techniques, and institutions that create, rationalize,
and sustain notions of difference and disparities. In contrast with the two
dominant approaches to health disparities that I described above, my focus
here is not on arguing about the existence, acceptability, or ethics of health
disparities, but on the ways that the notions of difference and disparities in
HIV/AIDS prevention are made meaningful by contingent structures, practices, and discourses (Fox 1999). In an increasingly transformative time, distinctions between healthy and unhealthy populations are rapidly dissolving
as everything becomes a potential hazard and everyone is seen as subject to
risk (Peterson 1997). In this way, constructs of HIV/AIDS risk and its underlying
causes leads to the privileging of particular types of behaviors and identities

over others (Fox 1999). The inequitable distribution of risk represents the productive power of differentiation and disparity, and their impact on subjectivities, especially in the field of HIV/AIDS prevention.

I am not arguing that current approaches to health disparities should no longer be considered. I am also not saying that it is better to simply understand notions of inequality and disparity as mere representations of broader transformations in governmentality, or to presuppose that they exist without much significant impact or consequence in determining and stabilizing the politics of difference. Instead, using the ethnographic evidence presented previous chapters, I contend that it is imperative to consider how various biomedical, public health, and social institutions and policies routinely naturalize various forms of difference. I also maintain that it is equally important to consider how recent transformations in commerce, biotechnology, and medicine have produced unstable and contradictory notions of what it is to be human—who we are, how we see ourselves, and how we relate to others. Here, I advocate for a broader reading of the institutions, practices, and discourses that make up health disparities. We need to realize and consider the extreme productive capacity and influence of health disparities, and the ways in which they ground and promote difference as an integral part of how we come to see and understand our health and society. Health disparities wield great influence over national social and economic agendas and public health practice, and they anchor individual and collective subjectivities in difference.

Health disparities are a powerful industry. They command considerable financial and administrative resources and enable the proliferation of various research and political agendas that keep intact categories of difference and the social and economic conditions that contribute to inequalities in health. In fact, the processes and discourses that make up health disparities have extensive vested interests, informing local, national, and international policy initiatives such as the US Healthy People 2020 initiative and the World Health Organization's goal of "Health for All";[8] funding and research; and the social contexts of lived experience.

Thus, health disparities have come to hold tremendous potential economic and political value. Disparities in health, as realized in the sociopolitical, scientific, and economic realms in which they have come to be engaged, are being made into social instruments of action by individuals and groups alike to secure political acknowledgment and to access forms of welfare benefits through the platform of social, economic, and biological difference. Those implicated within the debates about health disparities and those deemed to be at high risk must also be understood through their productive actions and choices in the name of inequitable burdens of affliction and illness.

The scope of health disparities is vast, extending into research, scholarship, policies, programs, and practices. Reducing health disparities, for instance, is a top priority for leading government agencies, and increasing percentages of federal and state health budgets have been appropriated for activities and services related to health disparities. Providers, patients, researchers, and policy makers also routinely collaborate to design health interventions and programs that are specifically tailored to accommodate racial, ethnic, and cultural differences. In Miami, prevention programs built as a result of disparities in HIV/AIDS are said to be keeping racial and ethnic minority populations alive. Therefore, not only have social differences become necessary and natural elements in the provision and design of health and health care, but they also serve as routine and normal ways in which we have come to understand the innate characteristics and disparities in health outcomes of individuals and groups.

Therefore, we need to take seriously the magnitude of the productive capacity of health disparities and the implications that this capacity has for various constituents in order to ameliorate the vast social inequalities that plague our country. The material realities and the enumerative practices that measure difference allow for the naturalization of health disparities—which means that difference and disparity come to stand as essential attributes of people, rather than an indication of a relationship between two groups. The policies and practices of health disparities sustain their potency by reproducing categories of difference and the very structures that contribute to inequalities in health. It is by attending to this productive capacity of health disparities that we might be able to think and act beyond the current boundaries of public health prevention measures that include biological treatments and behavioral and educational interventions, and push beyond solutions that are leveled at the social determinants of health—the underlying conditions of health inequities rooted in geopolitical, economic, and social forces. Current HIV/AIDS prevention measures and commitments to act on the social determinants of health do very little to alter the categories of difference, their social histories, and their rationalities that ground and perpetuate inequalities in health. We must act seriously and thoroughly to transform the sustainability and potency of these categories of difference if we are to move forward in improving people's daily lives.

6

Treating the West

Afterthoughts on Future Directions

Conceived by the Global Programme on AIDS at the World Health Organization (now called the Joint United Nations Programme on HIV/AIDS, or UNAIDS), World AIDS Day—December 1—was first observed in 1998. It is celebrated annually to remember those who have died, to show support for those living with HIV/AIDS, and to encourage unity in the fight against HIV/AIDS. In 2005 the theme for World AIDS Day was "Stop AIDS: Keep the Promise." A series of World AIDS Day events were organized in Miami to highlight the unequal impact of the epidemic on black residents. These included a special luncheon at Miami General Hospital, a day-long celebration at the city's convention center, and a series of marches in Liberty City—an area whose residents are predominantly impoverished African Americans and Haitian and that, according to the county's health department, has the highest number of cumulative AIDS and HIV cases in the county (Miami-Dade County Health Department 2007). A committee made up of members from local community-based organizations primarily serving black communities in Miami was responsible for organizing these events. I took part in the committee's meetings for a period of three months and attended all three events.

At the celebration at the convention center, health officials and event organizers framed the unequal burden of HIV/AIDS on black and African American communities nationwide and in Miami through the rhetoric of personal and social accountabilities. Activists commended the resiliency of those who were living with HIV/AIDS, and clients recounted stories of personal triumph through representations of cellular statistics. For instance, Terry Smith, a high-ranking official at the Miami-Dade County Health Department, focused his speech on the World AIDS Day theme by arguing that the notion of "promise" symbolized "accountability" and "personal responsibility." He explained that the goal of "keeping the promise" was "not only aimed at political leaders but also every individual person." He quoted Kofi Annan, then secretary general of the United Nations, saying that "all of us should make AIDS our problem" to point to the responsibility that we all had to fight HIV/AIDS, and he asked each of us in the audience to take the "opportunity to educate those around you" so that we would all be involved in raising awareness about the global effects of HIV/AIDS and the stigma that accompanies the disease. Terry Smith continued: "We have much to be thankful for in terms of accomplishments. The perinatal decline in AIDS was a huge marker of success and a great hope for women and children. Last year, only two cases of perinatal infection were reported in Miami. Florida has one of the most aggressive testing and counseling programs in the country. We test more people than other states." He paused as if to reflect, before declaring: "I encourage all of you to pray for a day when there will be a vaccine. I don't want this job forever, because I want to see a cure soon."

He further expressed pride in new and innovative programs spearheaded by the county health department—such as the black AIDS task force, the Latino AIDS task force, and the Florida black AIDS network—that were designed to reduce infection rates among racial and ethnic minority populations. He ended his speech by indicating that local governing bodies were very concerned about "implementing the national health disparities goals locally" and that they had ensured that in the past six years, the number of HIV/AIDS cases among blacks and African Americans had decreased by 28 percent in Miami-Dade County and by 30 percent in Florida overall.

Terry Smith reiterated notions embodied by the "we all have AIDS" campaign discussed in the opening vignette of this book. He reminded us about the universal accountability and responsibility that we all had in fighting HIV/ AIDS worldwide and encouraged all of us to "make AIDS our problem." At the same time, he outlined the accomplishments of his department in reducing the vast disparities in HIV/AIDS rates in Florida. These accomplishments included the fragmentation of programs, task forces, and networks by racial and ethnic groupings. He depicted notions of change, control, and success through the decreasing numbers of perinatal infections and the state's "aggressive" testing programs, while at the same time alluding to an ideal future when vaccine cures would eliminate the need for preventive services.

At the World AIDS Day luncheon at Miami General Hospital, which was sponsored by pharmaceutical companies, providers joined patient activists and clients in calling for progress in HIV/AIDS treatment and prevention and in celebrating those living with HIV/AIDS. Much like Terry Smith's illustrations of the successes of the county health department's initiatives, clients recited poems and stories of their miraculous transformations from sickness to vitality using the rhetoric of universal responsibility and individual accountability to describe personal achievements.[1] Community activists applauded these clients as "leaders" who truly embodied the notion of "positivity" because they demonstrated hope and perseverance in the midst of physical hardship. A young Haitian activist emphatically told the members of the audience: "Being HIV-positive means life, not death!" The audience gave him a standing ovation. Providers also joined in, praising clients and reminding them to be informed, aware, and knowledgeable about their medical care and risk for disease. For instance, one social worker encouraged clients to always keep "questioning why we can't do better in the field of HIV/AIDS," while giving a series of statistics about current rates of HIV/AIDS in Miami. Despite this rhetoric of encouragement and support, no one mentioned the vast disparities in HIV/AIDS rates, morbidity, and stigma that exist in Miami, nor did they discuss the severe economic, social, and political marginalization that undergird the daily lives of most of those in the room.

Although these events were organized against the backdrop of focusing attention on the universal responsibility for fighting HIV/AIDS worldwide and on what many, including the Centers for Disease Control and Prevention (CDC), label as an "HIV/AIDS crisis" among black and African American communities, they were not well attended. Even some of those confirmed on the agenda as expected to attend, including local politicians, community leaders, providers, and clients, failed to show up. Officials of the county health department attending the event at the convention center departed after Terry Smith's presentation of the department's accomplishments in reducing local rates of racial and ethnic health disparities in HIV/AIDS. After their departure, only about twenty people were left at the event although well over four hundred people had confirmed that they would attend it. The mayor and various council members also failed to show, although they were mentioned as primary speakers in the programs, and none of the organizers explained their absences to audience members. Fellow volunteers at the event surmised that this lack of official attention was due to what they called "racial tension," indicating that the organizers had been black and worked for community organizations that served black communities, while top officials in Miami were either Hispanic or white.

This sentiment was echoed by a handful of residents who attended a march in Liberty City. Only four people marched. One of them was the march organizer, a local resident. When she was asked about her motivation for holding the march, she replied: "Do you see any candlelight services in Liberty City? We have the highest percentages of AIDS cases in the community but who is having a rally here? No one!" (quoted in Berggren 2005). Using HIV/AIDS surveillance data, this resident pointed to the disconnect between the high rates of HIV/AIDS among African Americans and the dearth of attention to their plight. She blamed political and health officials for not acknowledging—through campaigns and public demonstrations such as the one that she organized—the vast numbers of African Americans and blacks who had died and who were still being affected by HIV/AIDS.

The HIV/AIDS luncheon at Miami General Hospital attracted many social workers, health educators, patient activists, and clients. But similar to the Liberty City march and the larger World AIDS Day event at the convention center, prominent physicians and other HIV/AIDS specialists, including the main speaker, who had promised to attend not only did not appear but also failed to give the organizers advance warning of their absence. I sat with the organizers for the luncheon, who were very upset by the turn of events and lamented the lack of prioritization of such events by leading providers. The mood was similar to that at the larger event at the convention center, where volunteer organizers suggested that racial tension was the reason why many leaders failed to attend and acknowledge the plight of so many black residents in Miami.

In addition, local media outlets neglected to report on local or national events related to World AIDS Day. When I tuned into the local news broadcasts at 5:00 P.M., 5:30 P.M., and 6:00 P.M., there was absolutely nothing about World AIDS Day—no mention of local, national, or global celebrations. There was instead a story about a bird that got stuck in a shipment of Christmas trees, and another one about an impending poinsettia shortage in Miami. At 11:00 P.M. there was a story—lasting about fifteen seconds—about a local World AIDS Day celebration in Fort Lauderdale.

The spirit and purpose of World AIDS Day and its theme of keeping the promise to make HIV/AIDS a collective problem represent the ideal of a unified global response and accountability. How this ideal is carried out in practice demonstrates the deep fragmentation—and the subsequent paradox—that exists in HIV/AIDS prevention in Miami and generally. The reality of the World AIDS Day events in Miami is that no one comes to them, and no one seems to care enough to devote any attention to the day. The lack of attention to and participation in these events is not new or surprising. Even though the official rhetoric consistently framed HIV/AIDS as an issue requiring a united response and as a major health concern for racial and ethnic minority populations in Miami, as shown through national and local surveillance data, the World AIDS Day events seem to represent just one of the many broader disconnects among official discourses of unified global response, community needs, and the on-the-ground practices they engender. These events also illustrate the ways in which concepts of social difference among populations and groups, particularly through notions of racial and ethnic health disparities, have become a normal and natural part of the political, social, and medical landscapes—so much so that public forums dedicated to addressing the persistent health disparities among black residents attract very little attention.

Divided Responsibility, Splintered Response

As Terry Smith did in his speech at the 2005 World AIDS Day event, public health institutions and governing bodies insist that they spend a significant portion of a continually decreasing amoung of HIV/AIDS funding on the African American community. They argue that they are following the dictates of the initiatives addressing national health disparities, implicitly maintaining that they are doing their part in alleviating health disparities and absolving themselves from any failures that result from these initiatives. The CDC and other federal agencies promise to increase resources for racially and ethnically tailored HIV/AIDS prevention programs—especially those aimed at African American and black communities—even though federal support of HIV/AIDS has continued to decline. For instance, the CDC stated that half of its HIV/AIDS prevention budget of $652 million and 63 percent of new funds were allocated to programs "designed for African Americans" in fiscal year 2007 (Centers for Disease Control and Prevention 2007b). In the following fiscal year, the CDC spent just under $369 million on prevention and research specifically targeted toward African Americans, or 49 percent of the overall budget for this purpose (Black AIDS Institute 2009). For fiscal year 2013 the CDC's budget for domestic HIV/AIDS prevention activities was $826 million, an increase of $40 million from the previous fiscal year (US Department of Health and Human Services 2012).

A large proportion of this increase is due to the focus on high-impact prevention approaches that are aligned with the 2010 National HIV/AIDS Strategy, the nation's first attempt to coordinate HIV/AIDS efforts. The strategy measures progress toward targets to be achieved by 2015, such as reducing new HIV infections and HIV-related health disparities and increasing access to care for people living with HIV/AIDS and improving their health outcomes (Office of National AIDS Policy 2010). Efforts are under way to implement the evidence-based programs that have demonstrated the greatest measurable success in reducing new HIV/AIDS infections in high-risk populations and geographic regions. Examples include large-scale testing initiatives like the Act against AIDS campaign, which delivers messages about testing targeted at specific groups at high risk for HIV infection (for example, "Take Charge. Take the Test" is designed for African American women, and "Testing Makes Us Stronger" is aimed at black men who have sex with men); individual behavioral interventions such as Women Involved in Life Learning from Other Women (WILLOW), which is designed for HIV-positive African American women and aims to provide education to increase gender pride, healthy social networks, and communication skills for discussing safe sex; and treatment as prevention, which has been proclaimed as transformational in the field of HIV/AIDS prevention because of its ability to improve clinical outcomes for HIV-positive individuals and its public health benefit in reducing the spread of infection.[2]

However, state and county health agencies highlight the fact that federal funding is continuously decreasing and vow to make up for these federal cuts in order to keep initiatives to reduce HIV/AIDS disparities functioning. They claim that HIV/AIDS prevention programs, like the racial and ethnic minority populations that they target, are being kept alive through state and county funding. For instance, the Florida Department of Health and the Miami-Dade County Health Department contend that they are apportioning funding to HIV/AIDS prevention programs aimed at racial and ethnic groups in spite of declining federal resources for HIV/AIDS. But in Florida in general, and especially in Miami, decreasing resources for HIV/AIDS efforts—particularly programs targeting racial and ethnic minority populations—have become the norm. At a 2006 meeting of the Miami-Dade HIV/AIDS Partnership, the official county planning board for HIV/AIDS, for instance, officials indicated that the county health department was going to absorb millions of dollars in funding cuts by the CDC and other federal agencies. By insinuating that they are doing all that they can in terms of funding allocation, federal, state, and local public health agencies absolve themselves from accountability and blame. If disparities in health continue to rise, then the culpability can easily be assigned to either inappropriate translations of programs at the local level or racial and ethnic minority populations themselves.

At the level of local health and social service organizations, administrators and directors spoke of dwindling funds and reductions in HIV/AIDS prevention programs for racial and ethnic minority groups, especially for efforts aimed directly at Haitians. At Sante Ayisyen, for example, the staff was exasperated at being unable to find funding for their fledgling clinical programs, pointing to donors who were seen as "out of touch" with the Haitian community by expecting more collaborations between competing organizations and being inflexible about local translations of certain evidence-based HIV/AIDS interventions. These were pressing issues for this organization, which—even with its ties to local research universities and the county health department—was struggling to meet demands in Little Haiti. In a similar predicament, Dr. Paul, the head of one of the few clinics catering to HIV-positive Haitians in Miami, was also being forced to merge his practice with Miami General Hospital, which meant that he could no longer see only his own patients.

Clients and activists also use narratives of racial and ethnic disparities to foreground and bolster local struggles to increase public awareness of and support for prevention programs directed at specific racial and ethnic groups. They employ complex strategies to live positively and formulate notions of responsible, ethical, and enlightened governance and citizenship, and they strive to fuse individual accountability with social responsibility. They extol the changes that were brought about by becoming HIV-positive status and that enable them to live as responsible citizens in control of their own health and well-being.

Patients portray their numerical subjectivity by their use of cellular-level statistics as markers of progress and meticulously document their CD4 levels and
T-cell counts. They use official surveillance data to call for greater allocations of
resources to communities in need and question why more has not been done to
ease the inequitable burden of disease.

However, as illustrated throughout this book, such configurations of subjectivity and governance are not easily translatable or sustainable for Haitians
in Miami, for whom such projects of social, political, and biological citizenship
always already embody racial and ethnic inequalities and discrimination. These
processes, although steeped in multiple gradients of power and authority, do
not completely render Haitians powerless or immobile. Haitians struggle to
produce alternative discourses and actions that challenge how HIV/AIDS prevention knowledge and practices operate and circulate. They refuse to tie themselves to official constructions of the management and mediation of risk, and as
a result they become positioned as difficult subjects and objects of governance.
By conceptualizing notions of HIV/AIDS, risk, and subjectivity through multiple
configurations of community and identity, Haitians in Miami turn structural
and social inequalities into broader issues of authority and social order. In this
way, Haitian clients remake HIV/AIDS prevention into a site not only of constant
struggles over knowledge production and meaning in science and public health,
but also of challenges to the rationalities of race, ethnicity, and culture through
everyday practices.

Chronicling HIV/AIDS at the Margins

The observation of World AIDS Day 2005 serve to bring the arguments outlined
in this book full circle. The science and practice of HIV/AIDS prevention advocate
for a type of response that mirrors the "we all have AIDS" campaign, in which we
all engage in a unified response to HIV/AIDS worldwide and think of ourselves
as at universal risk for HIV/AIDS. But the response of HIV/AIDS prevention on
the ground—influenced by surveillance practices, enumerative strategies, the
products of experts, and health disparities initiatives—fragments people into
categories of social difference and behavioral risk and acts on the vast disparities in HIV/AIDS morbidity and mortality through these same groupings. Official
discourses of HIV/AIDS no longer implicitly or explicitly deliberate the existence
of health disparities based on racial and ethnic differences. Instead, the CDC,
local departments of health, providers, scholars, activists, and clients focus on
how to alleviate the inequitable burden of illness that deeply affects many racial
and ethnic minority communities.

Particularly in Miami the notions of difference and disparity and the rhetoric of universal accountability and risk in the field of HIV/AIDS prevention
efforts have become more widespread. Techniques of enumeration, especially

those of HIV/AIDS surveillance, are foundational to how we come to know and act on populations and diseases. Experts and the public hail enumerative data as an authoritative and holistic representation of the epidemic and use the products of these data—calculations, maps, charts, and so forth—to call for a unified global response in the fight against HIV/AIDS. However, the daily practices of enumeration are highly dynamic, constantly shifting, and in a continual process of standardization. Triangulation allows the practices of standardization to enable seemingly fluid and self-evident translations of various structural and social inequalities into comparable and discrete categories, while simultaneously claiming that these products represent real and factual maps of the epidemic. Thus, enumerative practices produce multiple categories of risk and identity, enhance and reproduce the work done by difference and disparity, and in general fragment our knowledge and view of HIV/AIDS and the people most affected by it. They also naturalize the associations among risk, race, ethnicity, and culture in both official and public discourses of HIV/AIDS, so that risk becomes the central way in which experts view clients and clients see themselves.

These shifting practices in how we understand risk and subjectivity are by no means controlled only by powerful institutions like the CDC or departments of health: enumerative processes of standardization, data making, and naturalization also involve the active and inactive participation of clients who are the objects of standardization. Many clients, like Mary Long, the woman in Dr. Cruz's class described in chapter 2, identify themselves with numerical subjectivities and prevention goals through categories of risk and difference, while HIV/AIDS institutions and experts construct them as "risky" or "nonrisky" subjects and citizens. Haitians who are targeted by HIV/AIDS prevention strategies continually negotiate official and unofficial discourses of HIV/AIDS risk and understand and embody risk not through numerical subjectivity, but as a continual state of being that affects us all. They refuse individual and expert management of risk and counter the divisions made by experts between social and personal risk. Haitians are well aware of notions of risk and individual responsibility, even though experts portray them as incompatible objects of statistical data and subjects of HIV/AIDS prevention. For Haitians, HIV/AIDS is part of an enduring legacy of political discrimination, economic marginalization, and social prejudice rooted in historical considerations of slavery and imperialism. Because of the persistent renderings of Haitians as natural carriers of disease, many Haitians understand HIV/AIDS through the rubric of universal risk and describe themselves in ways that are distinct from numerical subjectivity.

Haitians navigate several realms of existence, as both productive and responsible citizens and as unmanageable subjects, even though HIV/AIDS experts position them as unsuitable objects of governance and subjects of expert mediation. In Miami HIV/AIDS experts locate risk and target interventions at the level of communities and their cultures. This link between culture and risk has shifted the notion of risk from a mainly biological and behavioral category to one that is associated with culture and embedded in ideological correlations between race and disease. In targeting prevention at the level of the community, HIV/AIDS experts and programs simultaneously dilute and concretize notions of community by conflating behavioral and biological traits with culture and community. Experts are continually urging Haitian clients to empower themselves and control their own medical destinies. But these experts' constructions of Haitians are entrenched in notions of social and biological primitivism and cultural baggage.

Haitian clients and advocacy groups also participate in both the circulation and the rejection of these discourses of HIV/AIDS, culture, and community. By conceptualizing HIV/AIDS through multiple frames of meaning—as something experienced, as a consequence of particular actions, and as a way to garner necessary resources—many Haitians challenge the epistemological foundations of HIV/AIDS risk reduction and prevention efforts. Their stories of health and illness become seen as illustrations of poverty, discrimination, and marginalization and disclose the myriad practices employed to navigate health and social service systems and government bureaucracies. Haitians are also entrenched in fractured notions of community and collective identity, as a result of the complex historical contexts of Haiti's sustained geographical, political, economic, and social isolation. By negotiating various diseases and institutions, Haitians challenge official narratives that position them and their risk for HIV/AIDS as overdetermined by culture.

Haitians in Miami also simultaneously assert and refuse positive living strategies, the fundamental components of HIV/AIDS prevention programs that stress empowerment, self-sufficiency, and medical compliance in the face of living with HIV/AIDS. Positive living is aligned with broader illness-based movements; gains traction through the production and management of responsible, ethical, and enlightened biological citizens; and is characterized by a set of biosocial practices that include safe sex, disclosure, and adherence to medication regimens. For many Haitians in Miami, such configurations of positive living do not hold together well, because these projects of biological citizenship are always already rooted in ideologies of racialized others, disease carriers, and unequal citizens. In their day-to-day negotiations with institutional bureaucracies and health and social service experts, Haitians highlight the politics of difference and exclusion embedded in the rationalities of positive living and biological citizenship.

Through various forms of participation and nonparticipation, Haitians continually separate themselves from biological conceptions despite official and popular renderings of them as carriers of risk and disease. Haitians have long been seen negatively as biological citizens in governmental policies, academic research, and popular culture. Strategies of positive living and biological citizenship minimize the continuing dominance of nationality, race, and other categories of social difference in citizenship discourses in the United States. As a result, these strategies overestimate the manipulability of life and the level of agency afforded to people with biological afflictions. Haitians and others who face the daily realities of poverty, social exclusion, and political marginalization may not reasonably possess the same desire or means for action in the name of biology.

Despite Haitians' attempts to decouple the associations of biology and citizenship, providers, policy makers, and the general public stress that HIV/AIDS prevention programs aimed at racial and ethnic minority groups are not only desirable but also necessary for the mediation of the inequitable burden of disease. These programs entrench categories of social difference and risk groupings into the daily practices of HIV/AIDS prevention and uphold the idea that race and ethnicity are foundational to the understanding of health disparities. Disparity and difference are relational terms in public health, meaning variation from the norm or established standard. In the field of HIV/AIDS prevention, however, the idea of disparity or difference is used and understood without this relational stance between two groups. In daily practice, difference and disparity now describe essential characteristics of individuals and groups. Discourses of Haitians and their poor health outcomes occur without the mention of a reference group for purposes of comparison. It is in these ways that health disparities have become natural and unquestioned components of our society, controlling significant material and social resources such as funding designations, social agendas, and national policy strategies. Health disparities are a powerful industry and enable various research and political strategies that sustain categories of difference and the root causes of health inequalities. Health disparities also play a significant role in positioning citizens as sources of value for the state. Individuals and groups also use difference and disparities to secure social and material benefits.

Moving Forward: Present and Future Reconsiderations

A thorough understanding of HIV/AIDS must be representative of interdisciplinary theoretical and methodological frameworks. It is only by critically engaging with theoretical approaches from medical anthropology, epidemiology, science and technology studies, critical race theory, and citizenship that I have been able to examine in detail how broader geopolitical structures, social norms, and local politics affect the daily lives of individuals and groups and the ways in which people come to understand and act on their own health and well-being. By working in sites of HIV/AIDS scientific and policy governance, prevention programs, and the social worlds of Haitians in Miami, I have also been able to observe the multiple ways in which HIV/AIDS prevention reproduces and naturalizes categories of difference and obscures and downplays the everyday suffering of the people it tries to know and act on. This book represents a body of work that uses these theoretical and methodological interventions to move beyond a sole focus on cultural interpretations or on the political economy of HIV/AIDS and to provide critical interpretations of the linkages among scientific knowledge, public health practice, community politics, and individual suffering.

HIV/AIDS prevention in the United States presents rich and highly relevant frames through which to explore contemporary issues related to the complex interplay between universal responsibility and social inequality. The paradox of HIV/AIDS prevention produces, sustains, and constantly reconfigures categories of difference and notions of disparity through the complex circulations of knowledge, discourses, and practices about HIV/AIDS and at-risk populations. It also illustrates the shifting and coproductive relationships among public health, biomedical science, and categories of people. Constructions of HIV/AIDS risk and prevention in the United States are still evolving. The CDC and local departments of health are continually developing and implementing various procedures of standardization in HIV/AIDS prevention strategies such as surveillance, testing, counseling, risk assessments, and treatment. New enumerative technologies like the Program Evaluation and Monitoring System and the Serological Testing Algorithm for Recent HIV Seroconversions, discussed in chapter 2, prove highly unstable in their role of interpreting and transmitting official representations of HIV/AIDS risk and categorizations of risky groups.

The discourse and practices of HIV/AIDS experts and officials are not solidified either. Health officials frequently problematize the feasibility of translating interventions into practice on the ground, and HIV/AIDS counselors convey uncertainty about the mediation of risk. In places such as Miami, these fissures in expert rationalities continually interface with Haitians' use of the various products of HIV/AIDS surveillance to negotiate subjectivities and reject expert mediation in the management of risk. Haitians continually construct, stifle, alter, appropriate, and question the science and practice of HIV/AIDS prevention, while officials position them as unsuitable objects of governance, risky subjects, and racialized others.

These everyday practices of HIV/AIDS prevention are highly dynamic, fragmented, and deeply contested. If we are to make critical changes in the study and practice of HIV/AIDS prevention in the United States, it is crucial that we shed presumed notions of unified "Western" or "American" HIV/AIDS prevention efforts, policies, experts, and lay publics. We must pay closer attention to the flexible and contested dynamics of HIV/AIDS prevention in the United States in medical, biotechnical, and policy settings and in the daily lives of those who reside in out-of-the-way global places like Miami.

HIV/AIDS prevention in the United States acquires its authority and potency by constructing HIV/AIDS as a medical, epidemiological, and social issue while simultaneously linking HIV/AIDS pathology to racial, ethnic, and immigrant identities. At a time when debates over race, science, and governance frequently occur in academic and public spheres, everyday practices of HIV/AIDS prevention programs underpin categories of individual and collective difference and sustain race and ethnicity as risk factors for HIV/AIDS. Scholars, providers, and clients further embed race and ethnicity as markers of risk by advocating for more specific groupings of difference, the development of programs aimed at specific racial and cultural groups, and the increased use of race and ethnicity in research to measure health disparities.

Categories of difference like race and ethnicity are central to how we come to understand HIV/AIDS prevention science and practice. They are also foundational to how we come to recognize and make sense of health disparities. The existence of health disparities is now taken for granted and seen as endemic to our society and no longer needing clarifications or deliberations. To be sure, health disparities are real and enduring forces that have profound structural and symbolic impact on individuals and communities. But we should not let the reality of disparities in health obscure the highly productive nature of the health disparities enterprise. If we are to mitigate the growing social and economic inequalities that affect us all, we must critically investigate how biomedical and public health science and practice contribute to the construction and maintenance of categories of difference as risk factors. As noted above, health disparities have become a powerful industry with a significant influence on funding priorities; global, national, and local policies; research initiatives; and lived experience. Health disparities have become significant ways in which we see ourselves and others in an increasingly globalized and fragmented world.

HIV/AIDS prevention programs, under the auspices of health disparities, make available critical resources to those who are designated as most vulnerable to poor health outcomes. Haitians—like many other racial, ethnic, and immigrant communities—negotiate various institutional programs and expert mediation to access resources that would otherwise unavailable to them. Haitians face severe social inequalities, political discrimination, and economic marginalization, and HIV/AIDS represents an economic and medical safety net in terms of cash subsidies and free medical care. Many Haitians assert social membership and citizenship claims through the platform of HIV/AIDS prevention. However, Haitians are not silent and willing subjects or objects of HIV/AIDS prevention. They continually produce, distort, appropriate, silence, and challenge the science and practice of HIV/AIDS prevention, making translations of HIV/AIDS prevention programming in Haitian communities difficult and, at times, nearly impossible.

Issues of political and economic marginalization, historical legacies of discrimination, and social constructions as racialized others are not addressed well, if at all, in the conceptualization and practice of HIV/AIDS programming. Failed translations and poor adoption of HIV/AIDS interventions by Haitian communities are often blamed on the culture and nature of Haitians themselves, who are seen as an uneducated group and as individuals overburdened by social and structural impediments. Public health policy and programs have to do better. They must look beyond purely genetic and biological approaches to HIV/AIDS and incorporate issues related to discriminatory policies concerning citizenship, debilitating economic marginalization, colonial and postcolonial historical contexts, and the social realities of lived experience. But even approaches that act on the social and structural determinants of health are not enough. Public health prevention must critically examine social and biological constructs of HIV/AIDS and at-risk populations and come to see and understand its own role in formulating and maintaining these constructs. Only in this way can public health prevention move beyond the policies and practices of inclusion and exclusion that ground HIV/AIDS programs today and begin to understand how people, like Haitians in Miami, are transforming and redefining what it means to suffer from the inequitable burden of disease at the margins. Individuals and groups affected by HIV/AIDS must be fully involved as equal partners for any solutions to be effective. By addressing their own authority, limitations, and culpability, those participating in HIV/AIDS prevention efforts and those affected by HIV/AIDS will be better equipped to face the enormous task of collaboratively designing practical solutions that are both meaningful and sustainable.

NOTES

CHAPTER 1   TREATING US, TREATING THEM

1. Following Paula Treichler (1999), I use "HIV/AIDS" to refer both to the epidemic that represents a wider social and cultural crisis and to the broad range of HIV-related clinical conditions—from asymptomatic infection to diseases used to define AIDS. At times I use HIV or AIDS alone, in conventional and accepted nomenclature like "HIV positive" or "AIDS prevalence."

2. Although I am acutely aware of the many opinions that exist about this nomenclature, to achieve consistency throughout the book, I have chosen to use the US Office of Management and Budget's standard racial and ethnic categories, especially in describing population estimates or in reporting information from government sources. In all government-related work, "black" or "African American" indicates individuals having origins in any of the black racial groups of Africa. In participant observation descriptions and interviews, I use "African American" to denote native-born Americans of African descent and "black" to denote those who are not native-born but are of African descent, including those from the Caribbean or Latin America.

3. Hispanics are 23 percent of Florida's adult population and account for 19 percent of the AIDS cases and 22 percent of the HIV infection cases in the state (Florida Department of Health 2011a).

4. These figures include only those who stated that they had been born in Haiti; people of Haitian descent who were born in the United States are not captured in this statistic but are subsumed under the African American category.

5. My work is directly aligned with Pigg's claim that public knowledge about HIV/AIDS in Nepal in the 1990s was being produced from prepackaged, established views of HIV/AIDS and prevention efforts. She writes: "Seen from the receiving end of this knowledge, however, and from the margins of its production, knowledge about AIDS and AIDS prevention does, however, come rather tightly packaged" (2001, 527n2).

6. I refer here to disciplines such as sociology, health psychology, and political science (see Parker 2001).

7. As criticisms of the structural reductionism of "center" versus "periphery" migration theories became more common, scholarship on transnationalism that focused on the complex partnerships between and tensions among states, global capital, and migrating populations gained credence (Braziel and Mannur 2003; Kearney 1995). Transnationalism represents ideas of connection, flexibility, and mobility across borders that were strengthened under late capitalism, as well as the multiple ways in which cultural flows and political and economic structures shape and influence the movement

of people, ideas, and objects (Appadurai 2008; Basch et al. 1994; Faist 2000; Glick Schiller 2004; Glick Schiller et al. 1992; Laguerre 1998; Ong 1999). Transnational communities, seen as dense networks across political borders created by immigrants in their quest for economic advancement and social and political recognition, represented ideas of connection, flexibility, and mobility across borders that, as noted above, were strengthened under late capitalism (Glick Schiller et al. 1992; Laguerre 1998; Ong 1999). Literature on transnationalism and diaspora also encompasses the emerging field of the anthropology of citizenship (Hann and Dunn 1996). Although citizenship is conventionally understood within the legal framework of modern democratic nation-states (Castles and Davidson 2000), analyses of transnationalism expand contexts of citizenship outside of the juridical sphere. They explore how, in addition to nation-states, various global institutions—such as transnational nonprofits, international organizations, and multinational corporations—today construct citizenship by employing various policies and practices; these policies and practices shape people's behavior in everyday life in specific ways in relation to certain objectives (Laguerre 1998; Ong 1999, 2003; Rose 1999; see also Foucault 2000).

8. I conducted fifty-three in-depth, semistructured interviews, each lasting from forty-five minutes to three hours. My interviewees were thirty-one Haitian and Haitian American clients who were accessing health services or who were HIV-positive, and twenty-two health and social service professionals working mainly with Haitian clients. Interviews with providers were conducted in English; interviews with clients were conducted in either Haitian Kreyòl or English, depending on the interviewee's preference. All interviews in Haitian Kreyòl were conducted with the aid of a Kreyòl-speaking translator, who helped clarify the more-complicated parts of the conversation. Provider interviews elicited data about relationships with Haitians identified as at high risk, assessments of the current field of HIV/AIDS research and services, and, in particular, the ways in which HIV/AIDS programs accommodate immigrant and minority communities. Interviews of Haitian clients elicited data about life experiences, conceptions of body and bodily processes, sex and sexual orientations, and health and illness. The documented themes related to understandings of HIV/AIDS; risk; identity; racism; and social, economic, and political barriers.

9. I conducted fieldwork at the Office of HIV/AIDS, one of the largest programs of the Miami-Dade County Department of Health. The office's initiatives included HIV prevention and education, patient care, the AIDS Drug Assistance Program, health education and risk reduction, counseling and testing services, and the Surveillance and Senior HIV Intervention Project. In addition, the office conducts professional training for healthcare workers, providers of counseling and testing services, volunteers wishing to work in health and social service agencies, and patient advocates. Over the course of several months, I was able to conduct both formal and informal interviews with key staff members and attend major educational training seminars on HIV/AIDS. This training was important not only because many institutions and professionals with whom I worked required that I become knowledgeable about and trained in HIV/AIDS issues in Florida and Miami-Dade County, but also because it gave me the opportunity to learn—as both a participant and an observer—how health and social service providers were trained. I also attended weekly meetings of the county's HIV/AIDS Partnership, the official county planning board for HIV/AIDS, and its various committees and subcommittees. The board is composed of health department administrators, community health workers, activists, and lay people, and its goal is to understand the ways in which different constituents develop and disseminate information related to

HIV/AIDS. As a result of my involvement with these different community coalitions and contacts from primary field sites, I was able to participate in and help plan community events related to HIV/AIDS, most of which centered on World AIDS Day 2006 and the National Black HIV/AIDS Awareness Day in February 2006.

10. My primary clinical field sites were Miami General Hospital and Sante Ayisyen (both pseudonyms). Miami General Hospital is one of the largest safety-net providers for the uninsured in Miami-Dade County, and one place where members of a majority of the county's medically impoverished immigrant communities receive care, including Haitians and Haitian Americans. It is also a leading center for HIV/AIDS care and treatment and, thus, participated in official discourses about HIV/AIDS through its clinical research. Miami General Hospital conducts weekly and biweekly educational classes on HIV/AIDS in English, Spanish, and Kreyòl for both patients and community members. Sante Ayisyen is a nonprofit community-based organization that provides health and social services to the underserved Haitian population of Miami. Its services include counseling, HIV testing, case management, assistance in buying food, health education, primary healthcare. It also conducts research and offers training and technical assistance to professionals in the social sciences and medicine. Because Sante Ayisyen is a key player in Haitian community politics and a vital provider of health and social services to underserved Haitians, conducting fieldwork here helped me better understand the concepts of community and identity through individual and institutional discourses. My other fieldwork sites included several health and social service organizations located in Little Haiti. These agencies were not only critical in providing services, but they also served as research and advocacy groups representing the Haitian community. I collaborated with providers from these agencies to gain a better understanding of the work done by and the community politics surrounding other Haitian community organizations. I also worked with providers from other larger agencies not located in Little Haiti and whose focus was not on the Haitian community per se in order to compare services for and outreach to other groups, particularly African Americans.

11. I spent half of my fieldwork time outside of clinical sites with my informants in a variety of settings—such as homes, churches, stores, and other similar locales—in order to better understand their daily lives in Miami. I worked closely with five key respondents over a fifteen-month period, spending the majority of time outside clinical settings. In drawing on people's narratives outside the clinic, I learned not only how people respond to HIV/AIDS prevention, but also about all of the other facets of their lives that interact with medical care.

12. I do not speak or understand Spanish well, so I do not know what was said in this situation. I also could not hear the tone of the voices and was unable to see facial expressions, as I was behind the men.

13. The neighborhood of Liberty City contains half of Miami-Dade County's African American population (US Bureau of the Census 2004). The riots began after an all-white jury acquitted four white police officers of violently beating and killing Arthur McDuffie, an African American insurance agent. The riots lasted about three days, killing eighteen people and causing millions of dollars in damage.

14. In both 1982 and in 1989, days of rioting occurred after a Hispanic police officer killed unarmed African American men.

15. In November 1980 an antibilingual initiative passed in Miami-Dade County, prohibiting any public expenditures involving non-English languages and non-US cultures. This legislation accompanied the Mariel boatlift, which brought into Miami younger

and poorer Cubans and mobilized Miami Cubans on local political issues. It was repealed in 1993.

16. This boycott was organized by African American leaders in Miami after local Cuban business and government leaders refused to give Nelson Mandela a key to the city during his visit in 1990, because of his ties to Fidel Castro. The boycott deepened tensions between African Americans and Cuban Americans and reduced the flow of tourist dollars into Miami.

17. François Duvalier was president and dictator of Haiti from 1957 until his death in 1971. His government became one of the most repressive in the world, marked by corruption and violence.

18. I will recount an experience here to buttress my claims about the critical importance of being established as a local. When I met the executive director of a local advocacy agency in Little Haiti, I introduced myself as a student from the University of California, San Francisco and Berkeley, who was studying health practices of Haitians in Miami. She responded by stating that she didn't understand why I was so far away from home, and why I wanted to work with them. Several days later, I returned with a letter from my "gatekeeper" on official University of Miami letterhead. After seeing this letter and having talked to my gatekeeper over the phone, she exclaimed, "Oh, you are from the University of Miami. Well. . . . I didn't know that. You should have said so in the first place. Welcome!" There is little doubt that UM is seen as a bastion of power, influence, wealth, and resources in the city of Miami, and in many ways, I would not have gained entry as smoothly without this affiliation.

CHAPTER 2   TREATING THE NUMBERS: HIV/AIDS
SURVEILLANCE, SUBJECTIVITY, AND RISK

1. Trudeau's book is very controversial. It claims that there are all-natural cures for common illnesses, chronic conditions, and infectious diseases such as HIV/AIDS. It also asserts that information about these all-natural cures is being suppressed by the government.

2. CD4 cells, or helper T-cells as they are sometimes called, are lymphocytes. About 15–40 percent of our white blood cells are lymphocytes, and they are important in protecting us from infections. CD4 cells serve as receptors to the HIV virus, enabling it to gain entry into the human body. Individuals' CD4 counts normally vary between 500 and 1,500 cells per cubic millimeter of blood. As HIV infection progresses, the number of these cells declines. The viral load is a measure of the amount of HIV virus in the bloodstream, expressed either as a number ranging from 48 to 10,000,000 copies/ml, or as the log of the viral load. The viral load affects the CD4 count, and a high load increases the risk of developing HIV infection or AIDS-related opportunistic infections. For somebody not on HIV treatment, a viral load above 100,000 is considered high, and one below 10,000 is considered low. When the CD4 count drops below 200 due to advanced HIV disease, a person is diagnosed with AIDS. Most people will experience an increase in CD4 cells and a decrease in viral load with effective HIV treatment.

3. A recent example of the complex and contested nature of HIV/AIDS surveillance occurred in 2007, when the Joint United Nations Programme on HIV/AIDS conceded that it had long overestimated HIV/AIDS rates globally and dropped the number of people with HIV/AIDS from 39.5 million to 33.2 million. This revelation highlighted

long-standing disputes among epidemiologists and other public health scholars on the validity of research methodologies used to arrive at such estimates (McNeil 2007).

4. PEMS data allow the CDC to monitor the adoption of evidence-based interventions and record details about the agencies implementing these interventions, characteristics of the populations targeted, and the locations and settings in which targeted populations are served.

5. Florida is one of the few states that identifies foreign-born populations in HIV/AIDS surveillance data. Florida classifies Haitians born in Haiti as "Haitian," and those born in the United States as "black/African-American."

6. In fact, even though Dr. Charles's organization was highly regarded among HIV/AIDS activists and academics, a few months after I left Miami in August 2006, its medical clinic closed and its HIV/AIDS social services system was completely shut down due to a lack of funding and political fallout. Similarly, another pivotal community-based organization that offered services to Haitians was in a state of crisis after its building suffered irreparable damage in Hurricane Rita, and that organization had to scramble to relocate and reestablish itself without much financial or logistical support. These instances are typical and reflect the precarious realities of both individual Haitians and organizations catering to Haitians in Miami.

7. The standards that are taught to counselors are those established by the CDC and include a "Counseling Model of Behavior Change," which is used to illustrate the ways in which counselors should personalize behavior change for their clients. This model is rooted in the premise that "behavior change cannot take place until the individual whose behavior needs changing takes ownership of his/her undesirable behavior, and change becomes significant to him/her" (Florida Department of Health 2005b, II-A-22).

CHAPTER 3   TREATING CULTURE: THE MAKING
OF EXPERTS AND COMMUNITIES

1. For further readings on the construction of credibility, see Epstein 1996.

2. SIDA is the Kreyòl word for AIDS, which is often referred to as maladi sida or sendwòm defisyans sistèm iminitè.

CHAPTER 4   TREATING CITIZENS: THE PROMISE OF POSITIVE LIVING

1. In 1997 Okaloosa AIDS Support and Informational Services founded the annual Positive Living Conference, considered to be one of the oldest and largest conferences for HIV-positive people.

2. There is a growing body of literature that critically engages with the scholarship on biological citizenship, biosociality, and, more broadly, the politics of life. See, for example, Sujatha Raman and Richard Tutton's (2010) careful analysis, using empirical work from science and technology studies, and Alexandra Plows and Paula Boddington's (2006) piece drawing on the body of work about green politics.

3. This was a common occurrence at Miami General, since much of the funding for HIV/AIDS intervention and prevention programs came from pharmaceutical companies.

4. A relatively recent example is an article in the Proceedings of the National Academy of Science (Gilbert et al. 2007) that states that the subtype B HIV virus in Haiti originated in Africa, and that Haiti—and, by implication, Haitians—were the conduit for the spread of HIV/AIDS to the Americas, including the United States. The authors' use

of various phylogenetic techniques, including bioinformatics and new cutting-edge sampling techniques, have won them support as well as criticism. There have been numerous reactions to the implications of this article, both positive and negative, from the scientific community and the public at large.

5. Haitians who do take classes sometimes choose the ones offered in English and sometimes the ones in Spanish.

6. As mentioned in chapter 1, in 1990 the Food and Drug Administration barred US blood banks from taking blood donations from Haitians because of the risk of contamination from HIV/AIDS. Although this ruling was repealed in December 1990 after massive protests by Haitians in the United States, it caused massive negative reverberations for Haitians living inside and outside the country (Pape 2000).

CHAPTER 5 TREATING THE NATION: HEALTH DISPARITIES AND THE POLITICS OF DIFFERENCE

1. See W. Anderson 2003; Barkan 1992; Cooper and David 1986; Gosset 1997; Gould 1981, 1994; Haller 1971; Haraway 1989; Harding 1993; Harris and Ernst 1999; F. Harrison 1995; King 1997; Krieger 1987; Omi and Winant 1994; Packard 1989; Reardon 2005; Shah 2001; Wailoo 1997; Whitmarsh and Jones 2010; D. Williams 1997.

2. Healthy People 2020 defines health equity as the "attainment of the highest level of health for all people. Achieving health equity requires valuing everyone equally with focused and ongoing societal efforts to address avoidable inequalities, historical and contemporary injustices, and the elimination of health and health care disparities" (US Department of Health and Human Services 2010).

3. Healthy People 2020 defines a health disparity as "a particular type of health difference that is closely linked with social, economic, and/or environmental disadvantage. Health disparities adversely affect groups of people who have systematically experienced greater obstacles to health based on their racial or ethnic group; religion; socioeconomic status; gender; age; mental health; cognitive, sensory, or physical disability; sexual orientation or gender identity; geographic location; or other characteristics historically linked to discrimination or exclusion" (US Department of Health and Human Services 2010).

4. According to Healthy People 2020, "the range of personal, social, economic, and environmental factors that influence health status are known as determinants of health. Determinants of health fall under several broad categories: policymaking, social factors, health services, individual behavior, biology, and genetics. It is the interrelationships among these factors that determine individual and population health. Because of this, interventions that target multiple determinants of health are most likely to be effective. Determinants of health reach beyond the boundaries of traditional health care and public health sectors; sectors such as education, housing, transportation, agriculture, and environment can be important allies in improving population health" (US Department of Health and Human Services 2010).

5. The Epidemiological Catchment Area Study focused on psychiatric disorders and concluded that low socioeconomic status strongly predicted higher risk for a varied number of psychiatric disorders (D. Williams and Collins 1995).

6. Assuming that a correlation at the population level applies at the individual level as well is commonly called an ecological fallacy.

7. There would be stratification within each category according to the other category (for example, gay African Americans), but those who identified as gay would not be categorized using the same parameters as those characterized by race or ethnicity.

8. In 1981 the World Health Assembly adopted the "Global Strategy for Health for All by the Year 2000." Its aim is not to eradicate all disease and disabilities but to ensure that resources for health are evenly distributed and that essential health care is available to all (World Health Organization 1981). This strategy was renewed in May 1998, with the adoption of the World Health Declaration by the Fifty-First World Health Assembly (World Health Organization 1998).

CHAPTER 6   TREATING THE WEST: AFTERTHOUGHTS
ON FUTURE DIRECTIONS

1. One of these poems and stories is discussed in the opening vignette in chapter 2.

2. In 2011 results from an international phase three clinical trial showed that sexual transmission of HIV/AIDS among heterosexual couples in which one partner is HIV-positive and the other is not was reduced by 96 percent with antiretroviral treatment (Cohen et al. 2011). Although extensive data have shown the preventive benefits of this treatment, this was the first randomized trial to demonstrate that clinical outcomes for individuals and transmission prevention could be markedly improved with treatment. In March 2012 the Panel on Antiretroviral Guidelines for Adults and Adolescents of the US Department of Health and Human Services updated its guidelines and recommended that antiretroviral therapy be initiated for everyone who has HIV, instead of waiting for evidence of severe immune suppression (US Department of Health and Human Services 2013).

REFERENCES

Allman, Timothy D. 1987. *Miami: City of the Future.* New York: Atlantic Monthly.

American Foundation for AIDS Research. 2006. "Kenneth Cole Launches Awareness Campaign." *Innovations,* summer, 1–9.

Anderson, Benedict. 1983. *Imagined Communities: Reflections on the Origin and Spread of Nationalism.* New York: Verso.

Anderson, John E., William D. Mosher, and Anjani Chandra. 2006. "Measuring HIV Risk in the U.S. Population Aged 15–44: Results from Cycle 6 of the National Survey of Family Growth." *Advance Data from Vital and Health Statistics* 377:1–27.

Anderson, Warwick. 2003. *The Cultivation of Whiteness: Science, Health and Racial Destiny in Australia.* New York: Basic.

Andrews, Stanley B. 1993. "Straight Sex and the Stigma of HIV/AIDS: Support Groups on the Gold Coast." *Practicing Anthropology* 15 (4): 33–36.

Appadurai, Arjun. 2008. "Global Ethnoscapes: Notes and Queries for a Transnational Anthropology." In *The Transnational Studies Reader: Intersections and Innovations,* edited by Sanjeev Khagram and Peggy Levitt, 50–63. New York: Routledge.

Baer, Hans, Merrill Singer, and Ida Susser. 1997. *Medical Anthropology and the World System: A Critical Perspective.* Westport, CT: Bergin and Garvey.

Bailey, Carol A. 2007. *A Guide to Qualitative Field Research.* 2nd ed. Thousand Oaks, CA: Pine Forge.

Banks, James, Michael Marmot, Zoe Oldfield, and James P. Smith. 2006. "Disease and Disadvantage in the United States and in England." *Journal of the American Medical Association* 295 (17): 2037–45.

Barkan, Elazar. 1992. *The Retreat of Scientific Racism: Changing Concepts of Race in Britain and the United States between the World Wars.* Cambridge, UK: Cambridge University Press.

Basch, Linda, Nina Glick Schiller, and Cristina Szanton Blanc. 1994. *Nations Unbound: Transnational Projects, Postcolonial Predicaments, and Deterritorialized Nation-States.* New York: Gordon and Breach.

Beck, Ulrich. 1992. *Risk Society: Towards a New Modernity.* Translated by Mark Ritter. London: Sage.

Becker, Howard S., and Blanche Geer. 1957. "Participant Observation and Interviewing: A Comparison." *Human Organization* 16 (3): 28–32.

Beine, David K. 2003. *Ensnared by AIDS: Cultural Contexts of HIV/AIDS in Nepal.* Kathmandu: Mandala Book Point.

Benton, Adia. 2012. "Exceptional Suffering? Enumeration and Vernacular Accounting in the HIV-Positive Experience." *Medical Anthropology* 31 (4): 310–28.

Berggren, Helen. 2005. "Taking a Stand against AIDS." *Miami Herald,* December 8.

Biehl, João. 2007. *Will to Live: AIDS Therapies and the Politics of Survival*. Princeton, NJ: Princeton University Press.

Biruk, Crystal. 2012. "Seeing Like a Research Project: Producing 'High-Quality Data' in AIDS Research in Malawi." *Medical Anthropology* 31 (4): 347–66.

Black AIDS Institute. 2009. "Making Change Real: The State of AIDS in Black America 2009." Accessed October 15, 2012. http://www.blackaids.org/reports/making-change-real.

———. 2011. "AIDS: 30 Years Is Enuf! The History of the AIDS Epidemic in America, 2011." Accessed October 15, 2012. http://www.blackaids.org/aids-30-years-is-enuf.

Bourgois, Philippe. 2000. "Disciplining Addictions: The Bio-Politics of Methadone and Heroin in the United States." *Culture, Medicine, and Psychiatry* 24 (2): 165–95.

———. 2003. "Crack and the Political Economy of Social Suffering." *Addiction Research and Theory* 11 (1): 31–37.

Bowker, Geoffrey C., and Susan Leigh Star. 1999. *Sorting Things Out: Classification and Its Consequences*. Cambridge, MA: MIT Press.

Braziel, Jana E., and Anita Mannur, eds. 2003. *Theorizing Diaspora: A Reader*. Malden, MA: Blackwell.

Briggs, Charles L. 2005. "Communicability, Racial Discourse, and Disease." *Annual Review of Anthropology* 34:269–91.

Briggs, Charles L., and Daniel C. Hallin. 2007. "Biocommunicability: The Neoliberal Subject and Its Contradictions in News Coverage of Health Issues." *Social Text* 25 (4): 43–66.

Briggs, Charles L., and Clara Mantini-Briggs. 2003. *Stories in the Time of Cholera: Racial Profiling during a Medical Nightmare*. Berkeley: University of California Press.

Brown, Karen M. 1991. *Mama Lola: A Voudou Priestess in Brooklyn*. Berkeley: University of California Press.

Butt, Leslie, and Richard Eves, eds. 2008. *Making Sense of AIDS: Culture, Sexuality, and Power in Melanesia*. Honolulu: University of Hawaii Press.

Cargill, Victoria A., and Valerie E. Stone. 2005. "HIV/AIDS: A Minority Health Issue." *Medical Clinics of North America* 89 (4): 895–912.

Carter-Pokras, Olivia, and Claudia Baquet. 2002. "What Is a 'Health Disparity?'" *Public Health Reports* 117 (5): 426–34.

Castles, Stephen, and Alastair Davidson, eds. 2000. *Citizenship and Migration: Globalization and the Politics of Belonging*. New York: Routledge.

Centers for Disease Control and Prevention. 1981. "Kaposi's Sarcoma and Pneumocystis Pneumonia among Homosexual Men—New York City and California." *Morbidity and Mortality Weekly Report* 30 (25): 305–8.

———. 1982. "Update on Acquired Immune Deficiency Syndrome (AIDS)—United States." *Morbidity and Mortality Weekly Report* 31 (37): 507–8, 513–14.

———. 1985. "Revision of the Case Definition of Acquired Immunodeficiency Syndrome for National Reporting—United States." *Morbidity and Mortality Weekly Report* 34 (25): 373–75.

———. 1986. "Current Trends Classification System for Human T-Lymphotropic Virus Type III/Lymphadenopathy-Associated Virus Infections." *Morbidity and Mortality Weekly Report* 35 (20): 334–39.

———. 1987. "Revision of the CDC Surveillance Case Definition for Acquired Immunodeficiency Syndrome." *Morbidity and Mortality Weekly Report* 36 (1S): 1–15.

———. 1989. "Current Trends Update: Heterosexual Transmission of Acquired Immunodeficiency Syndrome and Human Immunodeficiency Virus Infection—United States." *Morbidity and Mortality Weekly Report* 38 (24): 423–24, 429–34.

————. 1992. "1993 Revised Classification System for HIV Infection and Expanded Surveil-lance Case Definition for AIDS among Adolescents and Adults." *Morbidity and Mortal-ity Weekly Report* 41 (RR-17): 1–19.

————. 1994a. "Current Trends Heterosexually Acquired AIDS—United States, 1993." *Morbid-ity and Mortality Weekly Report* 43 (09): 155–60.

————. 1994b. "Current Trends Update: Impact of the Expanded AIDS Surveillance Case Defi-nition for Adolescents and Adults on Case Reporting—United States, 1993." *Morbidity and Mortality Weekly Report* 43 (09): 160–61, 167–70.

————. 1999. "Guidelines for National Human Immunodeficiency Virus Case Surveillance, Including Monitoring for Human Immunodeficiency Virus Infection and Acquired Immunodeficiency Syndrome." *Morbidity and Mortality Weekly Report* 48 (RR-13): 1–28.

————. 2001. "A Method for Classification of HIV Exposure Category for Women without HIV Risk Information." *Morbidity and Mortality Weekly Report* 50 (RR-06): 31–40.

————. 2005. "Office of Minority Health." Atlanta, GA: Centers for Disease Control and Pre-vention. Accessed April 24, 2005. http://www.cdc.gov/omh (site no longer contains information).

————. 2007a. "About Minority Health." Atlanta, GA: Centers for Disease Control and Pre-vention. Accessed June 6, 2007. http://www.cdc.gov/omhd/AMH/AMH.htm.

————. 2007b. "A Heightened National Response to the HIV/AIDS Crisis among African Americans." Atlanta, GA: Centers for Disease Control and Prevention. Accessed June 6, 2008. http://www.cdc.gov/hiv/topics/aa/resources/reports/heightendresponse.htm.

————. 2007c. "HIV/AIDS among African Americans." Atlanta, GA: Centers for Disease Con-trol and Prevention. Accessed June 6, 2008. http://www.hvtn.org/pdf/aa_fact_sheet .pdf.

————. 2008. "Revised Surveillance Case Definitions for HIV Infection among Adults, Adolescents, and Children Aged <18 Months and for HIV Infection and AIDS among Children Aged 18 Months to <13 Years—United States, 2008." *Morbidity and Mortality Weekly Report* 57 (RR-10): 1–8.

————. 2009. *Diagnoses of of HIV Infection and AIDS in the United States and Dependent Areas, 2007.* Vol. 19 of *HIV Surveillance Report.* Atlanta, GA: Centers for Disease Control and Prevention. Accessed June 27, 2013. http://www.cdc.gov/hiv/pdf/statistics_2007_HIV _Surveillance_Report_vol_19.pdf.

————. 2010. *Establishing a Holistic Framework to Reduce Inequities in HIV, Viral Hepatitis, STDs, and Tuberculosis in the United States.* Atlanta, GA: Centers for Disease Control and Prevention.

————. 2012. "Office of Minority Health and Health Equity." Atlanta, GA: Centers for Disease Control and Prevention. Accessed October 16, 2012. http://www.cdc.gov/minorityhealth/ OMHHE.html.

————. 2013a. *Diagnoses of HIV Infection and AIDS in the United States and Dependent Areas, 2011.* Vol. 23 of *HIV Surveillance Report.* Atlanta, GA: Centers for Disease Control and Prevention. Accessed July 29, 2013. http://www.cdc.gov/hiv/pdf/statistics_2011_HIV _Surveillance_Report_vol_23.pdf.

————. 2013b. "Statistics Center." Atlanta, GA: Centers for Disease Control and Prevention. Accessed July 25, 2013. http://www.cdc.gov/hiv/topics/surveillance/index.htm.

Clarke, Adele, Janet K. Shim, Laura Mamo, Jennifer R. Fosket, and Jennifer R. Fishman. 2003. "Biomedicalization: Technoscientific Transformations of Health, Illness, and U.S. Biomedicine." *American Sociological Review* 68 (2): 161–94.

Cohen, Myron S., et al. 2011. "Prevention of HIV-1 Infection with Early Antiretroviral Ther-apy." *New England Journal of Medicine* 365:493–505.

Colin, Jessie M., and Ghislaine Paperwalla. 2008. "People of Haitian Heritage." In *Transcultural Health Care: A Culturally Competent Approach*, 3rd ed., edited by Larry D. Purnell and Betty J. Paulanka, 231–47. Philadelphia: F. A. Davis.

Commission on Social Determinants of Health. 2008. *Closing the Gap in a Generation: Health Equity through Action on the Social Determinants of Health*. Geneva: World Health Organization. Accessed June 26, 2013. http://whqlibdoc.who.int/publications/2008/9789241563703_eng.pdf.

Comstock, R. Dawn, Edward M. Castillo, and Suzanne P. Lindsay. 2004. "Four-Year Review of the Use of Race and Ethnicity in Epidemiologic and Public Health Research." *American Journal of Epidemiology* 159 (6): 611–19.

Cooper, Richard, and Richard David. 1986. "The Biological Concept of Race and Its Application to Public Health and Epidemiology." *Journal of Health Politics, Policy and Law* 11 (1): 97–116.

Coreil, Jeannine, and Gladys Mayard. 2006. "Indigenization of Illness Support Groups in Haiti." *Human Organization* 65 (2): 128–39.

Creed, Gerald. 2004. "Constituted through Conflict: Images of Community (and Nation) in Bulgarian Rural Ritual." *American Anthropologist* 106 (1): 56–70.

Croucher, Sheila L. 1997. *Imagining Miami: Ethnic Politics in a Post-Modern World*. Charlottesville: University Press of Virginia.

Crush, Jonathan, Bruce Frayne, and Miriam Grant. 2006. *Linking Migration, HIV/AIDS, and Urban Food Security in Southern and Eastern Africa*. Washington: International Food Policy Research Institute. Accessed October 15, 2012. http://programs.ifpri.org/renewal/pdf/UrbanRural.pdf.

Cusick, Linda, and Tim Rhodes. 1999. "The Process of Disclosing Positive HIV Status: Findings from Qualitative Research." *Culture, Health, and Sexuality* 1 (1): 3–18.

Douglas, Mary. 1966. *Purity and Danger: An Analysis of Concepts of Pollution and Taboo*. London: Routledge.

Douglas, Mary, and Aaron Wildavsky. 1982. *Risk and Culture: An Essay on the Selection of Technical and Environmental Dangers*. Berkeley: University of California Press.

Dumit, Joseph. 2003. *Picturing Personhood: Brain Scans and Biomedical Identity*. Princeton, NJ: Princeton University Press.

Dworkin, Shari L. 2005. "Who Is Epidemiologically Fathomable in the HIV/AIDS Epidemic? Gender, Sexuality, and Intersectionality in Public Health." *Culture, Health, and Sexuality* 7 (6): 615–23.

Ember, Melvin, Carol R. Ember, and Ian Skoggard, eds. 2005. *Encyclopedia of Diasporas: Immigrant and Refugee Cultures around the World*. 2 vols. New York: Springer.

Engels, Friedrich. 1950. *The Condition of the Working-Class in England in 1844*. With a preface written in 1892. Translated by Florence Kelley Wischnewtzky. London: Allen and Unwin.

Epstein, Steven. 1996. *Impure Science: AIDS, Activism, and the Politics of Knowledge*. Berkeley: University of California Press.

———. 2003. "Inclusion, Diversity, and Biomedical Knowledge-Making: The Multiple Politics of Representation." In *How Users Matter: The Co-Construction of Users and Technologies*, edited by Nelly Oudshoorn and Trevor Pinch, 173–90. Cambridge, MA: MIT Press.

———. 2010. "Beyond Inclusion, Beyond Difference: The Biopolitics of Health." In *What's the Use of Race? Modern Governance and the Biology of Difference*, edited by Ian Whitmarsh and David S. Jones, 63–87. Cambridge, MA: MIT Press.

Espinoza, Lorena, H. Irene Hall, Felicia Hardnett, Richard M. Selik, Qiang Ling, and Lisa M. Lee. 2007. "Characteristics of Persons with Heterosexually Acquired HIV Infection, United States 1999–2004." *American Journal of Public Health* 97 (1): 144–49.

Fairchild, Amy L., and Ellen A. Tynan. 1994. "Policies of Containment: Immigration in the Era of AIDS." *American Journal of Public Health* 84 (12): 2011–22.

Faist, Thomas. 2000. *The Volume and Dynamics of International Migration and Transnational Social Spaces.* Oxford: Oxford University Press.

Fanon, Franz. 1967. *Black Skin, White Masks.* Translated by Charles L. Markham. New York: Grove.

Farmer, Paul. 1992. *AIDS and Accusation: Haiti and the Geography of Blame.* Berkeley: University of California Press.

———. 1999. *Infections and Inequalities: The Modern Plagues.* Berkeley: University of California Press.

———. 2003. *Pathologies of Power: Health, Human Rights, and the New War on the Poor.* Berkeley: University of California Press.

Farmer, Paul, and Didi Bertrand. 2000. "Hypocrisies of Development and the Health of the Haitian Poor." In *Dying for Growth: Global Inequality and the Health of the Poor,* edited by Jim Y. Kim, Joyce V. Millen, Alec Irwin, and John Gershman, 65–90. Monroe, ME: Common Courage.

Farmer, Paul, Margaret Connors, Kenneth Fox, and Jennifer Furin. 1996. "Rereading Social Science." In *Women, Poverty, and AIDS: Sex, Drugs, and Structural Violence,* edited by Paul Farmer, Margaret Connors, and Janie Simmons, 147–206. Monroe, ME: Common Courage.

Farmer, Paul, and Jim Y. Kim. 1991. "Anthropology, Accountability, and the Prevention of AIDS." *Journal of Sex Research* 28 (2): 203–21.

Fassin, Didier. 2007. *When Bodies Remember: Experiences and Politics of AIDS in South Africa.* Translated by Amy Jacobs and Gabrielle Varro. Berkeley: University of California Press.

———. 2009. "A Violence of History: Accounting for AIDS in Post-Apartheid South Africa." In *Global Health in Times of Violence,* edited by Barbara Rylko Bauer, Linda Whitford, and Paul Farmer, 113–35. Santa Fe, NM: School of American Research Press.

Fitzpatrick, John. 1981. "Reflections on Being a Complete Participant." In *Readings for Social Research,* edited by Theodore C. Wagenaar, 118–29. Belmont, CA: Wadsworth.

Florida Department of Health. 2002. "HIV Prevalence Estimates, Florida, 2002." Tallahassee: Florida Department of Health. Accessed October 1, 2007. http://www.doh.state.fl.us/disease_ctrl/aids/trends/prevalence/preves to2.pdf.

———. 2003. "HIV/AIDS among Haitians in Florida, Cumulative through December 2003." Tallahassee: Florida Department of Health. Accessed October 1, 2007. http://www.doh.state.fl.us/disease_ctrl/aids/updates/facts/2003HaitianFS.pdf.

———. 2004a. "HIV/AIDS in Florida's Haitian Population, 2004." Tallahassee: Florida Department of Health. Accessed October 1, 2007. http://www.doh.state.fl.us/Disease_ctrl/aids/updates/facts/04HaitianFact.pdf.

———. 2004b. "Risk Identification of HIV/AIDS Cases in Florida." Tallahassee: Florida Department of Health. Accessed October 1, 2006. http://www.doh.state.fl.us/disease_ctrl/aids/trends/slides/NIRs03.pdf.

———. 2005a. "Florida HIV/AIDS Annual Report/ Epidemiologic Profile 2005." Tallahassee: Florida Department of Health. Accessed October 1, 2007. http://www.doh.state.fl.us/disease_ctrl/aids/trends/epiprof/aids05.pdf.

———. 2005b. "Participant's Guide for HIV Prevention Counseling, Testing, and Referral Course [HIV/AIDS 501] and Prerequisite Course [HIV/AIDS 500]." Tallahassee: Florida Department of Health.

———. 2006a. "Impact of HIV/AIDS on Blacks and Hispanics by Country of Birth, 2005." Tallahassee: Florida Department of Health. Accessed October 1, 2007. http://www.doh.state.fl.us/Disease_Ctrl/aids/trends/slides/cob_live_05.ppt.

———. 2006b. "Out in the Open: The Continuing Crisis of HIV/AIDS among Florida's Men Who Have Sex with Men." Tallahassee: Florida Department of Health. Accessed May 1, 2008. http://www.doh.state.fl.us/disease_ctrl/aids/MSM_10_15_07.pdf.

———. 2010. "HIV Disease: United States vs. Florida." Tallahassee: Florida Department of Health. Accessed October 15, 2012. http://www.doh.state.fl.us/disease_ctrl/aids/updates/facts/10Facts/2010_US_VS_FL_Fact_Sheet.pdf.

———. 2011a. "Florida Annual Report 2011: Acquired Immune Deficiency Syndrome and Human Immunodeficiency Virus." Tallahassee: Florida Department of Health. Accessed October 15, 2012. http://www.doh.state.fl.us/disease_ctrl/aids/trends/epiprof/HIVAIDS_annual_morbidity_2011.pdf.

———. 2011b. "HIV among the Haitian-Born in Florida." Tallahassee: Florida Department of Health. Accessed July 29, 2013. http://www.doh.state.fl.us/disease_ctrl/aids/updates/facts/11Facts/2011_Haitians_Fact_Sheet.pdf.

Fordham, Graham. 2004. *A New Look at Thai AIDS: Perspectives from the Margin.* New York: Berghahn.

Fordyce, Lauren. 2008. "Birthing the Diaspora: Technologies of Risk among Haitians in South Florida." PhD diss., University of Florida.

Foucault, Michel. 1977. *Discipline and Punish: The Birth of the Prison.* Translated by Alan Sheridan. New York: Pantheon.

———. 1978. *The History of Sexuality.* Vol. 1: *An Introduction.* Translated by Robert Hurley. New York: Pantheon.

———. 1979. "On Governmentality." *Ideology and Consciousness* 6 (Autumn): 5–22.

———. 1991. *Remarks on Marx: Conversations with Duccio Trombadori.* Translated by R. James Goldstein and James Cascaito. New York: Semiotext(e).

———. 2000. *Power.* Edited by James D. Faubion and Paul Rabinow, translated by Robert Hurley. New York: New Press.

———. 2003. *Society Must Be Defended: Lectures at the Collège de France, 1975–1976.* Edited by Mauro Bertani and Alessandro Fontana, translated by David Macey. New York: Picador.

Fox, Nick. J. 1999. "Postmodern Reflections on 'Risk,' 'Hazards,' and Life Choices." In *Risk and Sociocultural Theory: New Directions and Perspectives,* edited by Deborah Lupton, 12–33. Cambridge: Cambridge University Press.

Frank, Emily. 2009. "Shifting Paradigms and the Politics of AIDS in Zambia." *African Studies Review* 52 (3): 33–53.

Franklin, Sarah, and Margaret Lock, eds. 2003. *Remaking Life & Death: Toward an Anthropology of the Biosciences.* Santa Fe, NM: School of American Research Press.

Frieden, Thomas R. 2010. "A Framework for Public Health Action: The Health Impact Pyramid." *American Journal of Public Health* 100 (4): 590–95.

Gamble, Vanessa N., and Deborah Stone. 2006. "U.S. Policy on Health Inequities: The Interplay of Politics and Research." *Journal of Health Politics, Policy and Law* 31 (1): 93–126.

Geertz, Clifford. 1973. *The Interpretation of Cultures: Selected Essays.* New York: Basic.

Giddens, Anthony. 1999. "Risk and Responsibility." *Modern Law Review* 62 (1): 1–10.

Gilbert, M. Thomas P., Andrew Rambaut, Gabriela Wlasiuk, Thomas J. Spira, Arthur E. Pitchenik, and Michael Worobey. 2007. "The Emergence of HIV/AIDS in the Americas and Beyond." *Proceedings of the National Academy of Sciences* 104 (47): 18566–70.

Gilman, Sander L. 1985. *Difference and Pathology: Stereotypes of Sexuality, Race, and Madness.* Ithaca, NY: Cornell University Press.

———. 1986. *Jewish Self-Hatred: Anti-Semitism and the Hidden Language of the Jews.* Baltimore, MD: John Hopkins University Press.

Ginsburg, Faye D., and Rayna Rapp, eds. 1995. *Conceiving the New World Order: The Global Politics of Reproduction.* Berkeley: University of California Press.

Glick Schiller, Nina. 1992. "What's Wrong with This Picture? The Hegemonic Construction of Culture in AIDS Research in the United States." *Medical Anthropology Quarterly* 6 (3): 237–54.

———. 2004. "Transnationality." In *A Companion to the Anthropology of Politics,* edited by David Nugent and Joan Vincent, 444–67. Malden, MA: Blackwell.

Glick Schiller, Nina, Linda G. Basch, and Christina Blanc-Szanton, eds. 1992. *Toward a Transnational Perspective on Migration: Race, Class, Ethnicity, and Nationalism Reconsidered.* New York: New York Academy of Sciences.

Goodman, Alan H. 2000. "Why Genes Don't Count (for Racial Differences in Health)." *American Journal of Public Health* 90 (11): 1699–702.

Goodwin-Gill, Guy S. 1996. "AIDS and HIV, Migrants, and Refugees: International Legal and Human Rights Dimensions." In *Crossing Borders: Migrants, Ethnicity, and AIDS,* edited by Mary Haour-Knipe and Richard Rector, 50–69. London: Taylor and Francis.

Gossett, Thomas F. 1997. *Race: The History of an Idea in America.* Oxford: Oxford University Press.

Gostin, Lawrence O., Scott Burris, and Zita Lazzarini. 1999. "The Law and the Public's Health: A Study of Infectious Disease Law in the United States." *Columbia Law Review* 99 (1): 59–128.

Gould, Stephen J. 1981. *The Mismeasure of Man.* New York: Norton.

———. 1994. "The Geometer of Race." *Discover,* November, 65–69.

Green, Thomas A. 1998. "Using Surveillance Data to Monitor Trends in the AIDS Epidemic." *Statistics in Medicine* 17 (2): 143–54.

Grenier, Guillermo J., and Alex Stepick. 1992. *Miami Now! Immigration, Ethnicity, and Social Change.* Gainesville: University Press of Florida.

Gros, Jean-Germain. 2000. "Haiti: The Political Economy and Sociology of Decay and Renewal." *Latin American Research Review* 35 (3): 211–26.

Gutmann, Matthew. 2007. *Fixing Men: Sex, Birth Control, and AIDS in Mexico.* Berkeley: University of California Press.

Hacking, Ian. 1982. "Biopower and the Avalanche of Printed Numbers." *Humanities in Society* 5 (3–4):279–95.

———. 1986. "Making Up People." In *Reconstructing Individualism: Autonomy, Individuality, and the Self in Western Thought,* edited by Thomas C. Hellner, Morton Sosna, and David E. Wellbery, 222–36. Stanford, CA: Stanford University Press.

Hader, Shannon L., Dawn K. Smith, Janet S. Moore, and Scott D. Holmberg. 2001. "HIV Infection of Women in the United States: Status at the Millennium." *Journal of the American Medical Association* 285 (9): 1186–92.

Hall, H. Irene, et al. . 2008. "Estimation of HIV Incidence in the United States." *Journal of the American Medical Association* 300 (5): 520–29.

Haller, John S. 1971. *Outcasts from Evolution: Scientific Attitudes of Racial Inferiority, 1859–1900.* Urbana: University of Illinois Press.

Hammett, Teresa A., Carol A. Ciesielski, Timothy J. Bush, Patricia L. Fleming, and John W. Ward. 1997. "Impact of the 1993 Expanded AIDS Surveillance Case Definition on Reporting of Persons without HIV Risk Information." *Journal of Acquired Immune Deficiency Syndromes and Human Retrovirology* 14 (3): 259–62.

Hann, Chris, and Elizabeth Dunn, eds. 1996. *Civil Society: Challenging Western Models.* London: Routledge.

Haour-Knipe, Mary, and Richard Rector, eds. 1996. *Crossing Borders: Migration, Ethnicity, and AIDS.* London: Taylor and Francis.

Haraway, Donna J. 1989. *Primate Visions: Gender, Race, and Nature in the World of Modern Science.* London: Routledge.

Harding, Sandra, ed. 1993. *The "Racial" Economy of Science: Toward a Democratic Future.* Bloomington: Indiana University Press.

Harper, Sam, John Lynch, Scott Burris, and George Davey Smith. 2007. "Trends in the Black-White Life Expectancy Gap in the United States, 1983–2003." *Journal of the American Medical Association* 297 (11): 1224–32.

Harris, Bernard, and Waltraud Ernst, eds. 1999. *Race, Science, and Medicine, 1700–1960.* London: Routledge.

Harrison, Faye V. 1995. "The Persistent Power of 'Race' in the Cultural and Political Economy of Racism." *Annual Review of Anthropology* 24:47–74.

Harrison, Kathleen McDavid, Tebitha Kajese, H. Irene Hall, and Ruiguang Song. 2008. "Risk Factor Redistribution of the National HIV/AIDS Surveillance Data: An Alternative Approach." *Public Health Reports* 123 (5): 618–27.

Hart, Jamie, and David R. Williams. 2009. *Toward Health Equity—The Cost of U.S. Health Disparities.* Ann Arbor, MI: Altarum Institute.

Harvey, David. 1989. *The Condition of Postmodernity: An Enquiry into the Origins of Cultural Change.* Cambridge, MA: Blackwell.

Haverkos, Harry W., and Raymond C. Chung. 2001. "AIDS among Heterosexuals in Surveillance Reports." *New England Journal of Medicine* 344 (8): 611–13.

Herdt, Gilbert, ed. 1997. *Sexual Cultures and Migration in the Era of AIDS: Anthropological and Demographic Perspectives.* New York: Oxford University Press.

Herdt, Gilbert, William Leap, and Melanie Sovine. 1991. "Introduction: Anthropology, Sexuality, and AIDS" *Journal of Sex Research* 28 (2): 167–69.

Hyde, Sandra T. 2007. *Eating Spring Rice: The Cultural Politics of AIDS in Southwest China.* Berkeley: University of California Press.

Jasanoff, Sheila, Gerald E. Markle, James C. Petersen, and Trevor Pinch, eds. 1995. *Handbook of Science and Technology Studies.* Thousand Oaks, CA: Sage.

Jenks, Angela C. 2010. "What's the Use of Culture: Health Disparities and the Development of Culturally Competent Health Care." In *What's the Use of Race? Modern Governance and the Biology of Difference,* edited by Ian Whitmarsh and David S. Jones, 207–24. Cambridge, MA: MIT Press.

Jones, Camara Phyllis. 2000. "Levels of Racism: A Theoretic Framework and a Gardener's Tale." *American Journal of Public Health* 90 (8): 1212–15.

Kahn, Jonathan. 2003. "Getting the Numbers Right: Statistical Mischief and Racial Profiling in Heart Failure Research." *Perspectives in Biology and Medicine* 46 (4): 473–83.

Kaiser Family Foundation. 2011. "Florida: Estimated Rates (per 100,000 Population) of AIDS Diagnoses, Adults and Adolescents, by Race/Ethnicity." Accessed October 15, 2012. http://kff.org/hivaids/state-indicator/aids-diagnosis-rate-by-re/.

———. 2013. "HIV/AIDS Epidemic in the United States." Menlo Park, CA: Kaiser Family Foundation. Accessed July 22, 2013. http://kff.org/hivaids/fact-sheet/the-hivaids -epidemic-in-the-united-states/.

Kalofonos, Ippolytos A. 2010. "All I Eat Are ARVs: The Paradox of AIDS Treatment Interventions in Central Mozambique." *Medical Anthropology Quarterly* 24 (3): 363–80.

Kaufman, Jay S., and Richard S. Cooper. 2001. "Commentary: Considerations for Use of Racial/Ethnic Classification in Etiological Research." *American Journal of Epidemiology* 154 (4): 291–98.

Kearney, Michael. 1995. "The Local and the Global: The Anthropology of Globalization and Transnationalism." *Annual Review of Anthropology* 24:547–65.

King, Gary. 1997. "The 'Race' Concept in Smoking: A Review of the Research on African Americans." *Social Science and Medicine* 45 (7): 1075–87.

Klevens, R. Monica, Patricia L. Fleming, Joyce J. Neal, and Jianmin Li. 1999. "Is There Really a Heterosexual AIDS Epidemic in the United States? Findings from a Multisite Validation Study, 1992–1995." *American Journal of Epidemiology* 149 (1): 75–84.

Kretsedemas, Philip. 2004. "Avoiding the State: Haitian Immigrants and Welfare Services in Miami-Dade County." In *Immigrants, Welfare Reform, and the Poverty of Policy*, edited by Philip Kretsedemas and Ana Aparicio, 107–36. Westport, CT: Praeger.

Krieger, Nancy. 1987. "Shades of Difference: Theoretical Underpinnings of the Medical Controversy on Black/White Differences in the United States, 1830–1870." *International Journal of Health Services* 17 (2): 259–78.

———. 1994. "Epidemiology and the Web of Causation: Has Anyone Seen the Spider?" *Social Science and Medicine* 39 (7): 887–903.

———. 2000a. "Counting Accountably: Implications of the New Approaches to Classifying Race/Ethnicity in the 2000 Census." *American Journal of Public Health* 90 (11): 1687–89.

———. 2000b. "Discrimination and Health." In *Social Epidemiology*, edited by Lisa Berkman and Ichiro Kawachi, 36–75. Oxford: Oxford University Press.

———. 2008. "Proximal, Distal, and the Politics of Causation: What's Level Got to Do with It?" *American Journal of Public Health* 98 (2): 221–30.

Krieger, Nancy, and Elizabeth Fee. 1994. "Man-Made Medicine and Women's Health: The Biopolitics of Sex/Gender and Race/Ethnicity." *International Journal of Health Services* 24 (2): 265–83.

Kumar, Chetan. 1998. *Building Peace in Haiti*. Boulder, CO: Lynne Rienner.

Kuntz, Diane. 1990. "Contagious Disease and Refugee Protection: AIDS Policy in the United States." *International Migration* 28 (3): 379–83.

Kutsche, Paul. 1998. *Field Ethnography: A Manual for Doing Cultural Anthropology*. Upper Saddle River, NJ: Prentice-Hall.

Laguerre, Michel S. 1984. *American Odyssey: Haitians in New York City*. Ithaca, NY: Cornell University Press.

———. 1998. *Diasporic Citizenship: Haitian Americans in Transnational America*. New York: St. Martin's.

Latour, Bruno. 1987. *Science in Action: How to Follow Scientists and Engineers through Society*. Cambridge, MA: Harvard University Press.

Latour, Bruno, and Woolgar, Steve. 1986. *Laboratory Life: The Construction of Scientific Facts*. 2nd ed. Princeton, NJ: Princeton University Press.

Lee, Benjamin, and Edward LiPuma. 2002. "Cultures of Circulation: The Imaginations of Modernity." *Public Culture* 14 (1): 191–213.

Lee, Philip R., Carroll L. Estes, and Fátima M. Rodriguez, eds. 2001. *The Nation's Health*. Sudbury, MA: Jones and Bartlett.

Leininger, Madeleine, ed. 1985. *Qualitative Research Methods in Nursing.* New York: Grune and Stratton.

Leshkowich, Anne Marie. 2007. "Circulation." Paper presented at the annual meeting of the American Anthropological Association, Washington, DC, November 28–December 1.

Levenson, Jacob. 2004. *The Secret Epidemic: The Story of AIDS in Black America.* New York: Pantheon.

Lindenbaum, Shirley. 1998. "Images of Catastrophe: The Making of an Epidemic." In *The Political Economy of AIDS,* edited by Merrill Singer, 33–58. Amityville, NY: Baywood.

———. 2001. "Kuru, Prions, and Human Affairs: Thinking about Epidemics." *Annual Review of Anthropology* 30:363–85.

Link, Bruce G., and Jo Phelan. 1995. "Social Conditions as Fundamental Causes of Disease." *Journal of Health and Social Behavior* 35 (Extra Issue): 80–94.

Lock, Margaret, Allan Young, and Alberto Cambrosio, eds. 2000. *Living and Working with the New Medical Technologies: Intersections of Inquiry.* Cambridge: Cambridge University Press.

Lockhart, Chris. 2008. "The Life and Death of a Street Boy in East Africa: Everyday Violence in the Time of AIDS." *Medical Anthropology Quarterly* 22 (1): 94–115.

Lorway, Robert, Sushena Reza-Paul, and Akram Pasha. 2009. "On Becoming a Male Sex Worker in Mysore: Sexual Subjectivity, 'Empowerment,' and Community-Based HIV Prevention Research." *Medical Anthropology Quarterly* 23 (2): 142–60.

Lupton, Deborah. 1999. "Introduction: Risk and Sociocultural Theory." In *Risk and Sociocultural Theory: New Directions and Perspectives,* edited by Deborah Lupton, 1–11. Cambridge: Cambridge University Press.

Lyttleton, Chris. 2000. *Endangered Relations: Negotiating Sex and AIDS in Thailand.* Bangkok: White Lotus.

MacLachlan, John. 1992. "Managing AIDS: A Phenomenology of Experiment, Empowerment and Expediency." *Critique of Anthropology* 12 (4): 433–56.

Mann, Jonathan M., Michael A. Grodin, Sophia Gruskin, and George J Annas, eds. 1999. *Health and Human Rights: A Reader.* New York: Routledge.

Marcelin, Louis H. 2005. "Identity, Power, and Socioracial Hierarchies among Haitian Immigrants in Florida." In *Neither Enemies nor Friends: Latinos, Blacks, Afro-Latinos/as,* edited by Anani Dzidzienyo and Suzanne Oboler, 209–27. New York: Palgrave.

Marcelin, Louis H., and Louise M. Marcelin. 2001. *Ethnographic Social Network Tracing among Haitian Immigrants in Miami.* Washington: Bureau of the Census.

Marcelin, Louis H., H. Virginia McCoy, and Ralph J. Diclemente. 2006. "HIV/AIDS Knowledge and Beliefs among Haitian Adolescents in Miami-Dade County, Florida." *Journal of HIV-AIDS Prevention in Children and Youth* 7 (1): 121–38.

Marmot, Michael, and Richard G. Wilkinson, eds. 1999. *Social Determinants of Health.* Oxford: Oxford University Press.

Marmot, Michael G., Manolis Kogevinas, and Mary A. Elston. 1987. "Social/Economic Status and Disease." *Annual Review of Public Health* 8:111–35.

Martin, Michèle A., Patricia Rissmiller, and Judy A. Beal. 1995. "Health-Illness Beliefs and Practices of Haitians with HIV Disease Living in Boston." *Journal of the Association of Nurses in AIDS Care* 6 (6): 45–53.

Matthews, Gene W., Verla S. Neslund, and R. Elliott Churchill. 1994. "Public Health Surveillance and the Law." In *Principles and Practice of Public Health Surveillance,* edited by Steven M. Teutsch and R. Elliott Churchill, 190–99. New York: Oxford University Press.

Matthews, Holly F. 2000. "Negotiating Cultural Consensus in a Breast Cancer Self-Help Group." *Medical Anthropology Quarterly* 14 (3): 394–413.

Mayfield Arnold, Elizabeth, Eugene Rice, Daniel Flannery, and Mary J. Rotheram-Borus. 2008. "HIV Disclosure among Adults Living with HIV." *AIDS Care* 20 (1): 80–92.

McDavid, Kathleen, and Matthew T. McKenna. 2006. "HIV/AIDS Risk Factor Ascertainment: A Critical Challenge." *AIDS Patient Care and STDs* 20 (4): 285–92.

McMichael, Anthony J. 1995. "The Health of Persons, Populations, and Planets: Epidemiology Comes Full Circle." *Epidemiology* 6 (6): 633–36.

McNeil, Donald G., Jr. 2007. "U.N. Agency to Say It Overstated Extent of H.I.V. Cases by Millions." *New York Times,* November 20.

Miami-Dade County Department of Planning and Zoning. 2007. "Persons of Haitian Ancestry or Ethnic Origin Who Were Counted in Census 2000 in Miami-Dade County 2000." Miami: Miami-Dade County Department of Planning and Zoning.

Miami-Dade County Health Department. 2007. "Miami-Dade County Neighborhood Profiles 2007." Miami: Miami-Dade County Health Department.

Mokotoff, Eve D., Lucia V. Torian, Monica Olkowski, James T. Murphy, Dena Bensen, Maree Kay Parisi, and Jennifer Chase. 2007. *CSTE Position Statement 07-ID-09: Heterosexual HIV Transmission Classification.* Atlanta, GA: Council of State and Territorial Epidemiologists. Accessed on July 26, 2013. http://c.ymcdn.com/sites/www.cste.org/resource/resmgr/PS/07-ID-09.pdf.

Mooney, Margarita. 2009. *Faith Makes Us Live: Surviving and Thriving in the Haitian Diaspora.* Berkeley: University of California Press.

Murray, Christopher J., Emmanuela E. Gakidou, and Julio Frenk. 1999. "Health Inequalities and Social Group Differences: What Should We Measure?" *Bulletin of the World Health Organization* 77 (7): 537–43.

Nachman, Steven R. 1993. "Wasted Lives: Tuberculosis and Other Health Risks of Being Haitian in a U.S. Detention Camp." *Medical Anthropology Quarterly* 7 (3): 227–59.

Nakashima, Allyn K., and Patricia L. Fleming. 2003. "HIV/AIDS Surveillance in the United States, 1981–2001." *Journal of Acquired Immune Deficiency Syndromes* 32 (Supplement 1): S68–85.

National Center for Health Statistics. 2001. "Healthy People 2000 Final Review." Hyattsville, MD: Public Health Service. Accessed October 15, 2012. http://www.cdc.gov/nchs/data/hp2000/ hp2k01.pdf.

National Women and AIDS Collective. 2008. "National AIDS Strategy for Women in the United States." New York: National Women and AIDS Collective. Accessed December 1, 2010. http://www.caear.org/downloads/09NWAC_NAS4women_transitionteam.pdf.

Navarro, Vincente, ed. 2000. *The Political Economy of Social Inequalities: Consequences for Health and Quality of Life.* Amityville, NY: Baywood.

———, ed. 2004. *The Political and Social Contexts of Health.* Amityville NY: Baywood.

Needle, Richard H., Richard T. Trotter, Merrill Singer, Christopher Bates, J. Bryan Page, David Metzger, and Louis H. Marcelin. 2003. "Rapid Assessment of the HIV/AIDS Crisis in Racial and Ethnic Minority Communities: An Approach for Timely Community Interventions." *American Journal of Public Health* 93 (6): 970–79.

Nelson, Diane M. 2009. *Reckoning: The Ends of War in Guatemala.* Durham, NC: Duke University Press.

Nguyen, Vinh-Kim. 2005. "Antiretroviral Globalism, Biopolitics, and Therapeutic Citizenship." In *Global Assemblages: Technology, Politics, and Ethics as Anthropological Problems,* edited by Aihwa Ong and Stephen J. Collier, 124–44. Malden, MA: Blackwell.

———. 2010. *The Republic of Therapy: Triage and Sovereignty in West Africa's Time of AIDS.* Durham, NC: Duke University Press.

Nguyen, Vinh-Kim, and Karine Peschard. 2003. "Anthropology, Inequality, and Disease: A Review." *Annual Review of Anthropology* 32:447–74.

Norris, Anne E., and Rosanna DeMarco. 2004. "The Mechanics of Conducting Culturally Relevant HIV Prevention Research with Haitian American Adolescents: Lessons Learned." *Journal of Multicultural Nursing and Health* 11 (1): 69–76.

Novick, Lloyd F., Cynthia B. Marrow, and Glen P. Mays. 2008. *Public Health Administration: Principles for Population-Based Management.* 2nd ed. Sudsbury, MA: Jones and Bartlett.

Office of National AIDS Policy. 2010. "National HIV/AIDS Strategy for the United States." Washington: White House. Accessed October 15, 2012. http://aids.gov/federal-resources/national-hiv-aids-strategy/nhas.pdf.

Okaloosa AIDS Support and Informational Services. 2007. "Positive Living." Accessed October 1, 2007. http://www.aidsoasis.org/PositiveLivingConference.html (site discontinued).

Omi, Michael, and Howard Winant. 1994. *Racial Formation in the United States: From the 1960s to the 1990s.* 2nd ed. New York: Routledge.

Ong, Aihwa. 1999. *Flexible Citizenship: The Cultural Logics of Transnationality.* Durham, NC: Duke University Press.

———. 2003. *Buddha Is Hiding: Refugees, Citizenship, and the New America.* Berkeley: University of California Press.

Owczarzak, Jill. 2009. "Defining HIV Risk and Determining Responsibility in Postsocialist Poland." *Medical Anthropology Quarterly* 23 (4): 417–35.

Packard, Randall M. 1989. *White Plague, Black Labor: Tuberculosis and the Political Economy of Health and Disease in South Africa.* Berkeley: University of California Press.

Pape, Jean W. 2000. "AIDS in Haiti: 1980–96." In *The Caribbean AIDS Epidemic,* edited by Glenford Howe and Alan Cobley, 226–42. Kingston, Jamaica: University of West Indies Press.

Pape, Jean W, Paul Farmer, Serena Koenig, Daniel Fitzgerald, Peter Wright, and Warren Johnson. 2007. "The Epidemiology of AIDS in Haiti Refutes the Claims of Gilbert et al." *Proceedings of the National Academy of Sciences* 105 (10): E13.

Pappas, Gregory, Susan Queen, Wilbur Hadden, and Gail Fisher. 1993. "The Increasing Disparity in Mortality between Socioeconomic Groups in the United States, 1960 and 1986." *New England Journal of Medicine* 329 (2): 103–9.

Parker, Richard. 2001. "Sexuality, Culture, and Power in HIV/AIDS Research." *Annual Review of Anthropology* 30:163–79.

Parker, Richard, and Peter Aggleton. 2003. "HIV and AIDS-Related Stigma and Discrimination: A Conceptual Framework and Implications for Action." *Social Science and Medicine* 57 (1): 13–24.

Patton, Cindy. 1985. *Sex and Germs: The Politics of AIDS.* Boston: South End.

———. 1990. *Inventing AIDS.* New York: Routledge.

Peterson, Alan. 1997. "Risk, Governance, and the New Public Health." In *Foucault, Health, and Medicine,* edited by Alan Peterson and Robin Bunton, 189–206. London: Routledge.

Petryna, Adriana. 2002. *Life Exposed: Biological Citizens after Chernobyl.* Princeton, NJ: Princeton University Press.

Pigg, Stacey Leigh. 2001. "Languages of Sex and AIDS in Nepal: Notes on the Social Production of Commensurability." *Cultural Anthropology* 16 (4): 481–541.

Pinkerton, Steven D., and Carroll L. Galletly. 2007. "Reducing HIV Transmission Risk by Increasing Serostatus Disclosure: A Mathematical Modeling Analysis." *AIDS and Behavior* 11 (5): 698–705.

Plows, Alexandra, and Paula Boddington. 2006. "Troubles with Biocitizenship?" *Genomics, Society, and Policy* 2 (3): 115–35.

Poovey, Mary. 1998. *A History of the Modern Fact: Problems of Knowledge in the Sciences of Wealth and Society*. Chicago: University of Chicago Press.

Porter, Theodore. 1995. *Trust in Numbers: The Pursuit of Objectivity in Science and Public Life*. Princeton, NJ: Princeton University Press.

Portes, Alejandro. 1997. "Immigration Theory for a New Century: Some Problems and Opportunities." *International Migration Review* 31 (4): 799–825.

Portes, Alejandro, and Alex Stepick. 1993. *City on the Edge: The Transformation of Miami*. Berkeley: University of California Press.

Prejean, Joseph, et al. 2011. "Estimated HIV Incidence in the United States, 2006–2009." *PLoS ONE* 6 (8): e17502.

PRNewswire. 2003. "Viacom and Kaiser Family Foundation Launch Comprehensive Initiative to Fight HIV/AIDS." *PRNewswire*, January 6. Accessed July 29, 2013. http://www .prnewswire.com/news-releases/viacom-and-kaiser-family-foundation-launch -comprehensive-initiative-to-fight-hivaids-73664642.html.

Quinn, Thomas C. 1994. "Population Migration and the Spread of Types 1 and 2 Human Immunodeficiency Viruses." *Proceedings of the National Academy of Sciences* 91 (7): 2407–14.

Rabinow, Paul. 1992. "Artificiality and Enlightenment: From Sociobiology to Biosociality." In *Incorporations*, edited by Jonathan Crary and Sanford Kwinter, 234–52. New York: Zone.

———. 1996. *Essays on the Anthropology of Reason*. Princeton, NJ: Princeton University Press.

———. 1999. *French DNA: Trouble in Purgatory*. Chicago: University of Chicago Press.

Raman, Sujatha, and Richard Tutton. 2010. "Life, Science, and Biopower." *Science, Technology, and Human Value* 35 (5): 711–34.

Raphael, Dennis. 2006. "Social Determinants of Health: Present Status, Unresolved Questions, and Future Directions." *International Journal of Health Services* 36 (4): 651–77.

Reardon, Jenny. 2005. *Race to the Finish: Identity and Governance in an Age of Genomics*. Princeton, NJ: Princeton University Press.

Rhatigan, Joe, Margaret Connors, and William Rodriguez. 1996. "Rereading Public Health." In *Women, Poverty, and AIDS: Sex, Drugs, and Structural Violence*, edited by Paul Farmer, Margaret Connors, and Jane Simmons, 207–44. Monroe, ME: Common Courage.

Robins, Steven. 2006. "'From Rights to Ritual': AIDS Activism and Treatment Testimonies in South Africa." *American Anthropologist* 108 (2): 312–23.

Rödlach, Alexander. 2006. *Witches, Westerners, and HIV: AIDS & Cultures of Blame in Africa*. Walnut Creek, CA: Left Coast.

Rogot, Eugene, Paul D. Sorlie, Norman J. Johnson, and Claudia Schmitt. 1992. "A Mortality Study of 1.3 Million Persons by Demographic, Social, and Economic Factors: 1979–1985 Follow Up." Bethesda, MD: National Institutes of Health.

Rose, Nickolas. 1999. *Powers of Freedom: Reframing Political Thought*. Cambridge: Cambridge University Press.

———. 2007. *The Politics of Life Itself: Biomedicine, Power, and Subjectivity in the Twenty-First Century*. Princeton, NJ: Princeton University Press.

Rose, Nikolas, and Carlos Novas. 2005. "Biological Citizenship." In *Global Assemblages: Technology, Politics, and Ethics as Anthropological Problems*, edited by Aihwa Ong and Stephen J. Collier, 439–63. Malden, MA: Blackwell.

Rosenberg, Charles. 1989. "What Is an Epidemic? AIDS in Historical Perspective." *Daedelus* 118 (2): 1–17.

———. 1992. *Explaining Epidemics and Other Studies in the History of Medicine.* Cambridge: Cambridge University Press.

Sangaramoorthy, Thurka. 2008. "Invisible Americans: Migration, Transnationalism, and the Politics of Difference in HIV/AIDS Research." *Studies in Ethnicity and Nationalism* 8 (2): 248–66.

———. 2012. "Treating the Numbers: HIV/AIDS Surveillance, Subjectivity, and Risk." *Medical Anthropology* 31 (4): 292–309.

Sangaramoorthy, Thurka, and Adia Benton. 2012. "Enumeration, Identity, and Health." *Medical Anthropology* 31 (4): 287–91.

Sangaramoorthy, Thurka, and Karen Kroeger. 2013. "Mobility, Latino Migrants, and the Geography of Sex Work: Using Ethnography in Public Health Assessments." *Human Organization* 72 (3): 263–72.

Satcher, David. 2006. "Ethnic Disparities in Health: The Public's Role in Working for Equality." *PLOS Medicine* 3 (10): e405.

Scheper-Hughes, Nancy. 1994. "AIDS and the Social Body." *Social Science and Medicine* 39 (7): 991–1003.

Serovich, Julianne M., Penny S. Brucker, and Jacob A. Kimberly. 2000. "Barriers to Social Support for Persons Living with HIV/AIDS." *AIDS Care* 12 (5): 651–62.

Setel, Phillip W. 1999. *Plague of Paradoxes: AIDS, Culture, and Demography in Northern Tanzania.* Chicago: University of Chicago Press.

Shah, Nayan. 2001. *Contagious Divides: Epidemics and Race in San Francisco's Chinatown.* Berkeley: University of California Press.

Shapin, Steven. 1995. "Here and Everywhere: Sociology of Scientific Knowledge." *Annual Review of Sociology* 21:289–321.

Shapin, Steven, and Simon Schaffer. 1985. *Leviathan and the Air-Pump: Hobbes, Boyle, and the Experimental Life.* Princeton, NJ: Princeton University Press.

Shim, Janet K. 2002. "Understanding the Routinised Inclusion of Race, Socioeconomic Status, and Sex in Epidemiology: The Utility of Concepts from Technoscience Studies." *Sociology of Health and Illness* 24 (2): 129–50.

Singer, Merrill. 1998. *The Political Economy of AIDS.* Amityville, NY: Baywood.

Singh, Gopal K., and Mohammad Siahpush. 2006. "Widening Socioeconomic Inequalities in US Life Expectancy, 1980–2000." *International Journal of Epidemiology* 35 (4): 969–79.

Smedley, Brian D., Adrienne Y. Stith, and Alan R. Nelson. 2003. "Introduction and Literature Review." In *Unequal Treatment: Confronting Racial and Ethnic Disparities in Health Care,* edited by Brian D. Smedley, Adrienne Y. Stith, and Alan R. Nelson, 29–79. Washington: National Academies Press.

Smith, George D. 2003. "Introduction: Lifecourse Approaches to Health Inequalities." In *Health Inequalities: Lifecourse Approaches,* edited by George D. Smith, xii–lix. Bristol, UK: Policy.

Smith, W. Shepherd, and Fred J. Payne. 1998. "Increasing Incidence of AIDS among Women." *Journal of the American Medical Association* 279 (5): 354–56.

Sobo, Elisa J. 1995. *Choosing Unsafe Sex: AIDS-Risk Denial among Disadvantaged Women.* Philadelphia: University of Pennsylvania Press.

Sohmer, Rebecca. 2005. *The Haitian Community in Miami-Dade: The Growing Middle Class Supplement.* Washington: Brookings Institute.

Star, Susan L. 1989. *Regions of the Mind: Brain Research and the Quest for Scientific Certainty.* Stanford, CA: Stanford University Press.

Star, Susan L., and James R. Griesemer. 1989. "Institutional Ecology, 'Translations,' and Boundary Objects: Amateurs and Professionals in Berkeley's Museum of Vertebrate Zoology, 1907–39." *Social Studies of Science* 19 (3): 387–420.

Starfield, Barbara. 2006. "State of the Art in Research on Equity in Health." *Journal of Health Politics, Policy and Law* 31 (1): 11–32.

Starr, Paul. 2009. "Professionalization and Public Health: Historical Legacies, Continuing Dilemmas." *Journal of Public Health Management and Practice* 15 (6 Supplement): S26–30.

Stepick, Alex.1992. "The Refugees Nobody Wants: Haitians in Miami." In *Miami Now! Immigration, Ethnicity, and Social Change*, edited by Guillermo Grenier and Alex Stepick, 57–82. Gainesville: University of Florida Press.

———. 1998. *Pride against Prejudice: Haitians in the United States*. Boston: Allyn and Bacon.

Stepick, Alex, Guillermo Grenier, Max Castro, and Marvin Dunn. 2003. *This Land Is Our Land: Immigrants and Power in Miami*. Berkeley: University of California Press.

Stepick, Alex, and Carol D. Stepick. 1990. "People in the Shadows: Survey Research among Haitians in Miami." *Human Organization* 49 (1): 64–77.

Stirratt, Michael J., Robert H. Remien, Anna Smith, Olivia Q. Copeland, Curtis Dolezal, Daniel Krieger, and the SMART Couples Study Team. 2006. "The Role of HIV Serostatus Disclosure in Antiretroviral Medication Adherence." *AIDS and Behavior* 10 (5): 483–93.

Strathern, Marilyn, ed. 2000. *Audit Cultures: Anthropological Studies in Accountability, Ethics, and the Academy*. London: Routledge.

Susser, Ida. 2009. *AIDS, Sex, and Culture: Global Politics and Survival in Southern Africa*. Chichester, UK: Wiley-Blackwell.

Thompson, Charis. 2005. *Making Parents: The Ontological Choreography of Reproductive Technologies*. Cambridge, MA: MIT Press.

Thornton, Robert J. 2008. *Unimagined Community: Sex, Networks, and AIDS in Uganda and South Africa*. Berkeley: University of California Press.

Treichler, Paula A. 1999. *How to Have a Theory in an Epidemic: Cultural Chronicles of AIDS*. Durham, NC: Duke University Press.

Trouillot, Michel-Rolph. 1990. *Haiti, State against Nation: The Origins and Legacy of Duvalierism*. New York: Monthly Review.

———. 1995. *Silencing the Past: Power and the Production of History*. Boston: Beacon.

Trudeau, Kevin. 2004. *Natural Cures "They" Don't Want You to Know About*. Hinsdale, IL: Alliance.

Tsing, Anna L. 2005. *Friction: An Ethnography of Global Connection*. Princeton, NJ: Princeton University Press.

US Bureau of the Census. 2004. *Ancestry 2000*. Washington: Department of Commerce.

———. 2010. *The Population with Haitian Ancestry in the United States: 2009*. Washington: Department of Commerce.

US Department of Health and Human Services. 1985. *Report of the Secretary's Task Force on Black and Minority Health*. Vol. 1: *Executive Summary*. Washington: Government Printing Office.

———. 1994. *Healthy People 2000*. 2nd ed. Washington: US Department of Health and Human Services.

———. 1999. "FY 2000 President's Budget for HHS." Washington: US Department of Health and Human Services. Accessed August 3, 2013. http://archive.hhs.gov/budget/fyo1budget/hhs2000.pdf.

———. 2001. *Healthy People 2010*. 2nd ed. Washington: US Department of Health and Human Services.

———. 2009. "Fiscal Year 2010 Budget in Brief." Washington: US Department of Health and Human Services. Accessed October 1, 2012. http://www.hhs.gov/about/budget/fy2010/fy2010bib.pdf.

———. 2010. "Healthy People 2020." Washington: US Department of Health and Human Services. Accessed October 1, 2012. http://www.healthypeople.gov/hp2020/.

———. 2011a. "About OMH." Washington: US Department of Health and Human Services. Accessed October 16, 2012. http://minorityhealth.hhs.gov/templates/browse.aspx?lvl=1&lvlID=7.

———. 2011b. "Healthy People 2020." Washington: US Department of Health and Human Services. Accessed July 22, 2013. http://www.healthypeople.gov/2020/GetInvolved/HealthyPeoplePresentation_2_24_11.ppt

———. 2012. "Fiscal Year 2013 Budget in Brief: Strengthening Health and Opportunity for All Americans." Washington: US Department of Health and Human Services. Accessed October 16, 2012. http://www.hhs.gov/budget/budget-brief-fy2013.pdf.

———. 2013. "Guidelines for the Use of Antiretroviral Agents in HIV-1-Infected Adults and Adolescents." Washington: US Department of Health and Human Services. Accessed July 24, 2013. http://aidsinfo.nih.gov/ContentFiles/AdultandAdolescentGL.pdf.

Valdiserri, Ronald O., Robert S. Janssen, James W. Buehler, and Patricia L. Fleming. 2000. "The Context of HIV/AIDS Surveillance." *Journal of Acquired Immune Deficiency Syndrome and Human Retrovirology* 25 (Supplement 2): S97–104.

Wadsworth, Michael E. 1997. "Health Inequalities in the Life Course Perspective." *Social Science and Medicine* 44 (6): 859–69.

Wailoo, Keith. 1997. *Drawing Blood: Technology and Disease Identity in Twentieth-Century America.* Baltimore, MD: John Hopkins University Press.

Whitmarsh, Ian, and David S. Jones. 2010. "Governance and the Uses of Race." In *What's the Use of Race? Modern Governance and the Biology of Difference,* edited by Ian Whitmarsh and David S. Jones, 1–23. Cambridge, MA: MIT Press.

Williams, David R. 1997. "Race and Health: Basic Questions, Emerging Directions." *Annals of Epidemiology* 7 (5): 322–33.

Williams, David R., and Chiquita Collins. 1995. "US Socioeconomic and Racial Differences in Health: Patterns and Explanations." *Annual Review of Sociology* 21:349–86.

Williams, David R., and James S. Jackson. 2000. "Race/Ethnicity and the 2000 Census: Recommendations for African American and Other Black Populations in the United States." *American Journal of Public Health* 90 (11): 1728–30.

Williams, Raymond. 1979. *Politics and Letters: Interviews with the New Left Review.* London: New Left.

Wood, Alastair J. 2001. "Racial Differences in the Response to Drugs-Pointers to Genetics Differences." *New England Journal of Medicine* 334 (18): 1393–96.

World Health Organization. 1981. "Global Strategy for Health for All by the Year 2000." Geneva: World Health Organization. Accessed July 29, 2013. http://whqlibdoc.who.int/publications/9241800038.pdf.

———. 1998. "World Health Declaration." Geneva: World Health Organization. Accessed July 29, 2013. http://www.nszm.cz/cb21/archiv/material/worldhealthdeclaration.pdf.

Young, Allan. 1982. "The Anthropologies of Illness and Sickness." *Annual Review of Anthropology* 11:257–85.

Zéphir, Flore. 1996. *Haitian Immigrants in Black America: A Sociological and Sociolinguistic Portrait.* Westport, CT: Bergin and Garvey.

Zierler, Sally, and Nancy Krieger. 1997. "Reframing Women's Risk: Social Inequalities and HIV Infection." *Annual Reviews of Public Health* 18:401–36.

INDEX

Page references to illustrations are in italics; page numbers followed by T indicate tables.

169

ABOUT THE AUTHOR

THURKA SANGARAMOORTHY is an assistant professor of anthropology at the University of Maryland, College Park, and a medical anthropologist who studies the relationships between the everyday lived experiences of individuals and communities and the biopolitics of global health institutions, neoliberal health policies, and enumerative practices. Her research and teaching interests are in the areas of medical anthropology, global public health, the anthropology of medicine, science and technology studies, HIV/AIDS, critical race theory, and citizenship. For more than ten years, Dr. Sangaramoorthy has conducted qualitative and ethnographic research in the fields of sexual health and the prevention of HIV and sexually transmitted diseases with vulnerable populations. She has worked with international nonprofits, state and local health departments, academic institutions, and governmental agencies to analyze public health policies related to health equity and the social determinants of health.

CPSIA information can be obtained at www.ICGtesting.com
Printed in the USA
BVOW03*1802100314

346948BV00001B/1/P